Case S

MW00783953

in Ethics, Diagnosis &
Treatment

Images of
Clients' Lives

Jeanmarie Keim, Ph.D., ABPP
with Kathleen Wells, Ph.D.

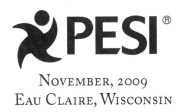

NOVEMBER, 2009
EAU CLAIRE, WISCONSIN

Published by:
PESI, LLC
PO Box 1000
3839 White Avenue
Eau Claire, Wisconsin 54702
Printed in the United States of America
ISBN: 978-0-9820398-7-8

PESI, LLC strives to obtain knowledgeable authors and faculty for its publications and seminars. The clinical recommendations contained herein are the result of extensive author research and review. Obviously, any recommendations for patient care must be held up against individual circumstances at hand. To the best of our knowledge any recommendations included by the author or faculty reflect currently accepted practice. However, these recommendations cannot be considered universal and complete. The authors and publisher repudiate any responsibility for unfavorable effects that result from information, recommendations, undetected omissions or errors. Professionals using this publication should research other original sources of authority as well.

For information on this and other PESI manuals and
audio recordings, please call 800-844-8260 or
visit our website at www.pesi.com

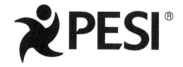

Dedication

To my daughter, Danielle, who teaches me about love;
And to all daughters with whom time is too brief

Acknowledgements

It is impossible to acknowledge all those who made this possible. Kate was my editor and coach, but more importantly my friend and colleague. She provided endless support, feedback, and encouragement from day one. My parents were supportive and provided childcare while I wrote. My mom read and gave feedback. My daughter said prayers and encouraged me each day.

Disclaimer

The cases in this book, while fictional, represent life events faced by people. While similarities may appear to exist between these fictional characters and actual people, the characters are fictional and any actual resemblance to any person is unintended and coincidental.

About the Authors

Jeanmarie Keim, Ph.D., ABPP, is a licensed psychologist and faculty member. She holds multiple degrees from Arizona State University. Currently, Jean is the Program Chair and trains counselors at the University of New Mexico. She is passionate about teaching, research and clinical work. Throughout many years in academia, Jean has taught diagnosis of mental disorders, ethics, psychotherapy theories, group procedures, group counseling, and group psychotherapy. She was recently elected as President-Elect of the Division of Group Psychology and Group Psychotherapy of the American Psychological Association. She is also active in the American Counseling Association. Jean has been nominated for excellence in teaching, received the 2009 President's Award for Outstanding Service to Division 49, APA, and received an American Indian Student Services Outstanding Faculty & Staff Award.

Kathleen Wells, Ph.D., is an Assistant Professor and Program Coordinator of the Family Studies and Human Development and Human Services degrees for the University of Arizona South. She is an editor and internationally published author. Her graduate work in anthropology and psychology plus over fifteen years of teaching supported her contributions to this text.

Table of Contents

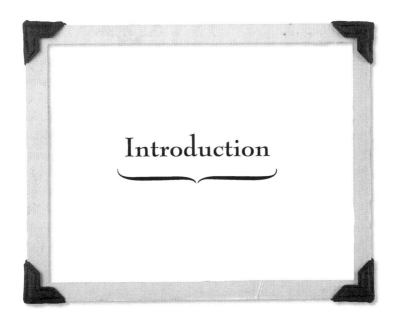

Introduction

Each of our lives has various events, images, or layers that, when combined, have immense impact on who we are. These cases provide images of the clients' lives, who they are, what they experience, and their feelings.

The cases that follow can be used to address many different course or self-study topics. Each case provides sufficient information and symptoms to diagnose one or more of the main characters. The cases may also be approached from various theoretical perspectives. For example, the reader of Frances could conceptualize the case from a psychodynamic, family, cognitive, behavioral, existential, or other theoretical perspective. Those readers focusing on ethics will find ethical issues present in each case. The ethical dilemmas give us the opportunity to reflect on how we would handle difficult decisions. Some readers will elect to address the three areas simultaneously; however, most readers will focus on one area at a time, returning to the case at a later date to consider the other areas.

Choosing whether to focus on diagnosis, theoretical case conceptualization, or ethics is easily accomplished. The ethical dilemmas do not interfere with diagnosing or conceptualizing the cases. Nor does the reader have to diagnose a character to envision a theoretically-based treatment for the character. While conceptualizing the cases, the ethical issue can be either taken into consideration as part of the conceptualization, or the ethical area could be set aside while conceptualizing treatment.

For Your Consideration

At the beginning of each case, there is a section entitled, "For Your Consideration." The reader is given elements to consider or reflect upon while reading the case. The elements are designed to help readers focus their attention on the most salient or critical aspects of the case.

Discussion Questions

Following each case is a group of discussion questions. Some focus on the case as a whole, while others focus on one of the three areas: diagnosis, theoretical approach, or ethics. Readers should select those questions that delve into the areas of their interest.

Pathology:

When examining the cases to determine diagnoses, the following approach is suggested: read the case and gain a sense of the client. Then re-read the case and identify any symptoms. Readers should group symptoms according to similarity and determine which general diagnostic category the symptoms fit within (mood, anxiety, eating, psychotic, etc.). Once a general diagnostic category for the symptoms is identified, determine which diagnosis might fit. Evaluate the symptoms against the diagnostic criteria and decide whether to assign that diagnosis. Finally, consider the overall stressors and functioning.

Theory:

Mental health professionals are encouraged to ground their clinical conceptualizations and treatment plans in theoretical statements that describe the etiology of mental health and illness. Most practitioners have a theoretical orientation, generally consisting of one theory or the combination of a couple theories that work well together. In this text, the readers are challenged to stretch beyond their theoretical orientations and consider the cases from multiple theoretical perspectives. The first step is to read the case and reflect upon it. Then, select a theoretical orientation from which to approach the case. Once the orientation is selected, the reader should consider what is going well for the client and what is not (i.e., the client's strengths and weaknesses). Consider where the client is in relation to developmental milestones. (Note, unless specifically mentioned in the case, the developmental milestones for each client were normal.) Psychosocial stages of the clients represented in the cases are important, in particular, with some theoretical orientations. Thus, many factors concerning the clients presented in the cases are critical and should be considered. Occasionally, the reader will have to make assumptions about the client's history because the information was not provided in the case study. It is important to note assumptions and proceed with the case based on these.

Once the above factors are considered in a case conceptualization, treatment goals and an initial treatment plan should be developed. If the reader has also elected to make a diagnosis(es), the diagnosis(es) will factor into the case conceptualization in a more concrete way. If the reader has not made a diagnosis, the conceptualization should focus more on symptoms, cognitions, defense mechanisms, etc. in formulating the conceptualization.

Ethics:

Each case has a summary of ethical and legal points to consider and there are discussion questions centering on the dilemmas. In reality, some of these concerns might necessitate a referral. When the focus is not on ethics, the reader is encouraged to assume the ethical issue is resolved and proceed accordingly with diagnosis and/or treatment. This is easily accomplished, as the ethical issue is only one aspect of the entire case. When reflecting on the ethical aspects of the case, the reader should consult the appropriate professional ethical codes and state statutes. Many alternatives exist for resolving the situations presented. A brief discussion of ethical issues follows each case. Consider what is best for the client rather than what meets the needs of the mental health professional when considering the appropriate course of action. Readers should note that ethics discussions following the cases center on the psychology, counseling, social work, and addictions professions. Citations in the text do not represent all codes nor are they an exhaustive list of the four codes represented in relation to the topic cited. Although every effort has been made to include those codes containing the ethical issues represented, readers should consult their professional codes in detail.

Case Studies:

It has been a journey to bring these clients to life, and to share images of their lives with others. They represent broad diversity in terms of ethnicity, socioeconomic status, abilities, geographic location, and age. What follows is a brief introduction to them.

Miguel is a young, Hispanic student residing on the south side of Tucson. His maternal grandparents, Alonzo and Maria, are retired migrant farm workers who reside with Miguel's family. Maria insisted their six children go to school when possible. Alonzo did not view education as a priority. Lupe, Miguel's mother, is their oldest daughter with whom they now reside. Lupe dropped out of high school to marry her life's love, Hector. Hector worked as an apprentice and learned the plumbing trade. He earns a good living, but does have many aches and pains from the hard physical work. He insists Miguel and his siblings not only get an education but also are very successful in school. Miguel struggles to balance the many layers of his life.

Frances is a 59-year-old Caucasian female. Her family of origin had a farm in the Imperial Valley. Frances believes it is no longer possible to compete with the large corporate farms, and that is what killed her father. Her mom is of sound mind; her health, however, is showing the years. Frances is one of three children. Peter was drafted and killed in Vietnam. John is 68 and works as an accountant. Frances is married and has children. She is struggling with her roles in life.

Linda Faith will be a Junior at the local high school in two weeks. She is Caucasian with blond hair and blue eyes. Linda Faith participates in activities and does well in school. Her parents are David, an attorney, and Michelle, who has a business degree. Linda Faith has a younger sister, Sarah Grace. Sarah Grace is very active in youth activities at a community center. Linda Faith's life consists of many demands and images that intertwine.

Samuel is a Navajo male who grew up in Northeastern Arizona and Northwestern New Mexico on the reservation. His parents are both Navajo and have always resided within twenty-five miles of where they were born. His mom, Wanda, is a weaver, and his father, Jack, is a construction worker. Samuel finished high school in May 1999 after which he trained and worked as a cook. Samuel has a strong sense of community. He struggles with the layers of family, community, work, and self.

Angela is a 37-year-old African American female. She attended Florida State University and earned her Bachelor's degree in Business with a Purchasing concentration. Angela has worked for about fifteen years as a Materials Manager for a firm that produces computer printers. She is responsible for ordering the parts, having them quality inspected, and getting them to the production line. Angela is reflecting on her personal and professional choices.

Sally is four. Her father has been employed in the construction industry for the past six years, and her mother works at home doing clothing alterations. Sally is an only child and her parents could not have been prouder. Being the first grandchild, she was probably photographed a thousand times, prior to leaving the hospital, and many thousands of photos were taken after that. Deciding to pursue treatment is a difficult decision, especially for the parents of this young girl.

Grant is a 35-year-old Caucasian male from a two-parent family. His father was a miner and his mother a schoolteacher. Both are now retired. He has two siblings. His older brother was the football star of the small Virginia mining town. His younger sister was Daddy's girl. Grant attended college near his hometown. After college he moved to Alaska to pursue a lucrative job with the oil companies. Grant is exploring how to fit the layers of his life together.

Yolanda is a young female from a poor family. She lives in Memphis and works as a prostitute. She was adopted when she was about four and was the oldest child in her adopted family. Her adoptive mother criticized her, complained about her behavior, and called her a liar. She dropped out of high school in tenth grade due to pregnancy. Yola is trying to balance working as a prostitute with being a single parent.

John is an eighteen-year-old Caucasian male who is experiencing difficulty at college. This is his first semester and his first time away from home. He came to the university counseling center because he is struggling with his classes. It is now Thanksgiving, and he is passing one out of four courses. John hesitated going away to college, due to the Virginia Tech and Illinois shootings before he graduated from high school. John is struggling with his new role as a college student.

Deborah is a 21-year-old college student, and Karen is her roommate. They share meals together and talk with each other. Deborah has always been very self-conscious and lacked confidence. She faces the financial pressures of attending college and has worked while in school. Deborah is a young woman working hard to balance all aspects of her life.

Roger is a thirty-year-old Caucasian male. He is the only son of his parents, who are of Jewish and German descent. His father was an astronomer and moved to the desert southwest to avoid light pollution as is found on the east coast. Roger completed high school and has successfully worked for a number of years as a salesman. He is married and currently stressed by the competing concerns he faces.

Lilly is a Hispanic female who recently retired from her clinical practice. She is in her mid-fifties. Lilly decided to volunteer in her local community by offering her services to disaster victims. This quickly became international work and she is always on the go. Lilly faces putting together the layers of her life.

Veronica is an attractive first generation American of Vietnamese heritage. Her parents fled on a small boat before the collapse of their county. Her family had some relatives in the U.S. who had left Vietnam a few months prior to the collapse who assisted them. They started an appliance repair shop that became profitable, and her family lives comfortably. Veronica has an older and a younger sibling, both brothers. The family has no religious affiliations. She is married to Greg, and they live in the San Fernando Valley. Veronica is trying to fit the pieces back together.

Hope is a forty-year-old, separated, single mom. She has four children with her estranged spouse. Hope works diligently to take care of her children. She has had many turns in her life creating various layers that she continues to face.

People often ask if these are real clients; the answer is no. They are merely images formed after many years of creating examples for teaching purposes. These images grew over the years and became the characters.

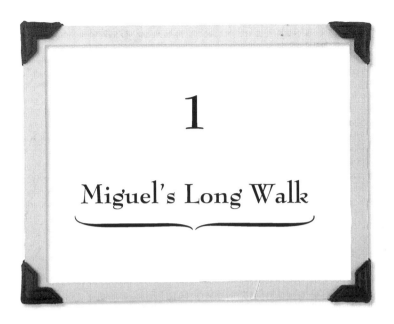

1

Miguel's Long Walk

For Your Consideration

As you read about Miguel and his experiences, be aware of your biases and how they impact your interpretation of the case. Consider whether a diagnosis is appropriate. Various treatment options exist, and could be provided by professionals from differing professional fields, for Miguel. Consider who would be best to provide treatment and why. Finally, what cultural and ethical issues are critical to address?

Miguel's Story

Miguel shifted his backpack yet again as he walked Charro Street toward the elementary school in south Tucson. Only seven o'clock in the morning, but the sun already baked the street and brought sweat to his face. His small, dark-haired sister, Maria, clung to his hand and held back, as she did every morning when he dropped her off at the playground. As the oldest boy, it was his responsibility to see her safely delivered to the teachers before continuing to his school. His fourteen-year-old sister, Ruth, walks with her friends now that she is a freshman at the high school.

Miguel stopped at the edge of a tall chain link fence. Children were already at play, parents and grandparents seeing them safely through the gates. "Come on, Maria. Time to go." He nudged her toward the gate.

"I don't want to." A pout filled her lips. "I want to go with you," she whined.

"We go through this every day. I have to go to high school. You have to go here."

"I want to go to high school." She stomped her little foot, hardening Miguel's resolve. He had decided a long time ago Maria got too much of her own way.

"You have to go through elementary, and then middle school, before high school. You'll get there before you know it. Now go on, Maria, get moving or we'll both be late." He gave her a firm push toward the gate and earned himself a nasty look. He chuckled which only made her angrier. He could see it in the look she was famous for. "Move it," he snapped, barely able to hide an affectionate smile.

She crossed her little arms and took on a stance he knew meant trouble. How was it he could be so smart at school, be the star forward on the soccer team, and his seven-year-old sister could wrap him around her finger and turn him to mush?

"Maria," he said in his most authoritative tone. "Go to school. Remember, Nana Maria will be very proud of you for going to school and learning well."

He glimpsed a look of pride as it slipped across her face before she hid it once more behind her stubborn streak. "I don't want to. It's boring to be here alone all day."

"You have lots of friends. Go on now. Go and play, then get to class. I'll see you this afternoon, little sister." Miguel smiled as he watched indecision flash across her face. She seemed to be deciding whether to fight.

Their gazes locked for a full minute, then apparently figuring out this was a battle she wouldn't win, Maria turned and stomped onto the playground. Spotting friends already at play, she bolted for the swing set, and Miguel knew her short-lived pout was done for the day.

He glanced at his watch, and then hurried down the sidewalk. At the corner he heard shrieking, and stopped to turn back for a last look. It always made him smile to see the little ones greeting each other as they were dropped off by their families. The school was the safest place in this part of town. The tall fence and security guards, discreetly watching the arrival of the students, ensured the children would be safe for the day.

Suddenly, a purple low-rider swung around the corner, the driver gunning its engine. The teen and two passengers were slumped low in the seat, but Miguel didn't need to see them. He knew the Impala. What the hell are they up to? he wondered. The car careened down the street going way too fast for the school zone. The crossing guard yelled at a half dozen kids and parents to hurry to the curb, just as the purple vehicle sped through the crosswalk. Miguel's heart seemed to stop then raced erratically. His breath caught in his throat as realization hit him. This was not good, not good at all. Those boys meant trouble.

As Miguel dove for cover behind some garbage cans, he saw a gun barrel aimed out of the open car window. Everything dropped to slow motion as a spray of bullets raked the terrified children and adults. The thunder of the shots was deafening as parents and grandparents threw themselves to the ground on top of their screaming children, trying desperately to keep them alive. Others bolted and ran for the building. Screams echoed in his mind, long after the noise of the gunfire faded. The car ripped around the corner not ten feet from his hiding place. Miguel held his breath; his heart pounded in his chest. A roar lingered in his ears as panic threatened to overtake him, and sweat broke out on his body and ran unchecked down his back. He prayed to Mother Mary the gang members in the car had not seen him. If they did, he'd be dead by night-fall.

When the sound of the car faded, he jumped up and looked frantically for Maria in the frightened crowd. The sight of two bodies, one young and one old splayed across the walk, blood running from multiple wounds sickened him. Guards already leaned over them, cell phones in hand, no doubt dialing 9-1-1.

Maria! He had to find her. Miguel thought of his parents, grand-parents, and siblings. If anything happened to Maria, it would break all of their hearts. She was his to protect. Where is she? Miguel's mind screamed. He scanned the terrified crowd and finally spotted Maria being hurried indoors with the other students. He knew the school would be locked down in seconds; he couldn't possibly get to her now, but at least he knew she was safe. Now he had to get away before someone found out he had witnessed the shooting. Miguel turned and ran from the deadly scene.

Four days later Miguel's mother, Lupe, cried softly into a tissue as she stood in the subdued interior of the funeral home. His father, Hector, and Miguel stood on either side of her gently supporting her between them. These were not the first gang related victims they had accompanied to the cemetery, and Lupe knew they would not be the last. She prayed every day for the safety of the children and those of the community, but it didn't seem to be helping. Was God not listening to her pleas?

Education was the key. She was sure of it. Her children had to learn and grow, and get away from the violence. They needed to live a better life than what they had here. Oh, she and Hector had tried to give them everything, but it wasn't enough. How could they give back life if it was lost to the gangs?

Two caskets were carried to the waiting hearses by strong young men, all nephews of her good friend, Socorro. She and her grand-daughter, Luisa, had perished in the drive-by shooting. The funeral mass had been long and sad. Such senseless violence was never easy to understand. Miguel was rigid beside her; not a tear fell down her son's face, as they did down Hector's. Miguel seemed made of stone. She lifted a hand to touch his cheek, but he jerked away from her touch. Maybe this hit him harder than any of them realized, she thought. Even though he'd been at his own school when it happened, the fact they knew the victims must have shaken him up. She would have Father Enrique speak with him. No matter how senseless, death was a part of life after all.

A gentle tap sounded on Miguel's bedroom door. "Miguel? Are you in there?" Ruth called out.

He thought about ignoring his sister, but knew she wouldn't give up. He lay on his bed, his hands behind his head with his fingers interlocked. "I'm here, pest. Come in."

The door slowly opened and she peeked around the edge. "Miguel, I need help."

His heart jumped. Had the gangs bothered her? He sat up and motioned her in. When she stepped around the door, he was relieved to see her math book. His breathing slowed to a normal pace and he took a deep breath. "Homework?"

She nodded and walked over to sit on the bed at his side.

"Then why didn't you say so?"

She shrugged. "I didn't want to bother you so soon after. . . well, you know."

"It's all right. We have to keep up with normal things to help with the terrible ones sometimes." He reached for the book she held. "So, what's the problem?"

A knock on the door interrupted her reply.

"Now who's there?" Miguel asked. Another head poked around the opening door. "Marco, come on in. We're having a convention."

"A what?" the boy asked.

"Never mind," Miguel grumbled. "What do *you* need?"

"Help with my English. My teacher says I am mixing Spanish words with the English, and I can't do that anymore. She said I have to decide which language I am using and stick with it." He sighed heavily as he plopped down on Miguel's other side.

Together they worked on math and English. Occasionally, Miguel's attention drifted and he became lost in thought. Ruth and Marco kept bringing him back to the subject of homework until finally they were almost done. Suddenly, a car backfired and Miguel pushed both kids to the floor as books and papers went flying. Ruth's breath whooshed out of her body when Miguel landed none too gently on top of her. Marco had the wind knocked out of him from hitting the floor so hard, but Ruth jumped to her feet.

"What's the matter with you? It was just a car!" She stooped to pull Marco to his feet, and then picked up her scattered papers and book.

"I'm sorry, Ruthie." Miguel shook his head. "I guess it just startled me. You two go on now. Finish up in your rooms."

As they were leaving, Miguel got up and went to the window to close it and lower the blind. His gaze ran up and down the street before he did so. There was no sign of the purple Impala, and he let out the breath he'd been holding as he approached the window.

"Miguel, it's hot in here. Why are you closing the window?"

"I don't like busybodies being able to see what I'm doing. *Ahora vayanse de aqui.* Go on now go away. Go do the rest yourselves."

With their heads hanging, his brother and sister left without another word. Miguel hated to hurt their feelings, but he knew they were safer in their own rooms than his. His was vulnerable on the street side of the house.

The Saturday after the funeral came around, and Miguel was grateful for a non-school day. Even if it meant yard work and chores, it was better than going to school. He had been approached again by the boys in the purple Impala. They seemed to be suspicious, but Miguel didn't think they had seen him. At least, he hoped and prayed they had not seen him.

In the garage, he bent over the lawn mower trying to figure out why the darned thing wouldn't start. He'd tuned it up recently, putting a new spark plug in it and changing the oil. That should have taken care of the problem. He twisted off the gas cap. Hmmm . . . full. He rocked back on his heels, lost in thought, wondering if they were going to need to take the machine to a repair place. A hand slapped onto his shoulder, and without thinking for even a split second, Miguel twisted and swung, catching his father right on the chin with his closed fist. Hector landed on his butt on the garage floor, shaking his head and swearing.

"Miguel! What on earth is wrong with you?"

Miguel was already scrambling to offer his hand to his dad. "Sorry, Papa. Are you all right?"

Hector slowly regained his feet, rubbing his chin and moving his jaw to be sure it still worked like it was supposed to. "I'm fine, but why are you so jumpy?"

"You snuck up on me." Miguel hung his head and failed to meet Hector's gaze.

"No, I didn't. I walked right in. I even called your name and you didn't answer, so I touched you."

"I'm sorry. I'll be more careful."

"Can't you tell me what's bothering you, son? Are the boys at school still teasing you about your academics and sports?"

Miguel shook his head. "No, Papa."

"You don't seem to be yourself these days. Your mother and I are worried."

"It's nothing. I'll work it out on my own." He clamped his jaw shut.

"Well, I suppose you're at the age when a man has to start taking care of his troubles himself." Hector smiled a bit, again touching his hand to his chin. "Well, I know I don't have to worry about you. You can take care of yourself. Now, tell me what is ailing this ancient piece of equipment?"

Five weeks later, Miguel walked down Calle Conejos. He'd been taking a new route to school since the shooting. This morning Mr. Sanchez, the bakery manager, called out a greeting, and Miguel listlessly responded as he continued walking. When he neared the corner he heard the sound of an engine he would recognize to his dying day. The Impala cruised around the corner and pulled up beside him. Sweat broke out on Miguel's forehead. What did they want with him? he wondered. Then he realized he'd known all along what they wanted. And he definitely didn't want what they did. How could he get out of this?

Miguel's cousin leaned toward the window. "*Hola*, Miguel. What's up with you?"

"*Nada*, Alejandro." Miguel forced the words around the lump in his throat and fought to slow the racing of his heart.

"We want to have a word with you."

"I got things to do, Cuz. I'll catch you later."

Alejandro frowned at him. "We're not going to ask again."

Miguel glanced into the car. On the backseat between two of the guys lay an automatic weapon. One of the boys followed Miguel's gaze, and then reached over to lay his hand on the high-powered gun.

"People are safer in *la familia* than outside. We don't think much of outsiders. Make your choice — in or out. We'll expect an answer after school today."

With that, they revved the engine and sped off, turning the corner on two wheels. Miguel realized he was shaking from the encounter. Did they know he had seen what they did? Were they determined to get him into the gang to control him? What am I going to do? Miguel wondered.

His decision made, Miguel turned and headed home. His parents weren't going to like it, but it was the only way he could stay alive.

Lupe glanced up as Miguel stepped through the back door and into the kitchen.

"What are you doing home, *mijo*? You should be at school. Don't you feel well?"

"I'm not going to school anymore, Mama. It is past time for me to go to work and help out around here."

Shocked by his statement, Lupe dropped onto a kitchen chair, wiped her hands carefully on a dishtowel as though gathering her thoughts. At last her gaze met Miguel's. "You are not going to drop out. We get by fine. Your grandmother, Maria, knows how important school is, and so do I."

"But *Tata* Alonzo always says having a good trade is more important than books, especially for the boys. Look at Papa. He's a plumber and he makes a fine living."

"Your grandparents worked hard picking lettuce and following the crops to support us. We even helped out in the fields when we were old enough to do it." She sighed. "I dropped out of school to marry *su padré* and have a family. I don't regret it, but for a woman that is bad enough, to rely on others to care for them. But for you, *mijo*, it is impossible! You will be trying to take care of a wife and children by flipping burgers some place. I won't have it!"

"I'm sorry, Mama. You have nothing to say about it. I'm not going back."

"But what about your sports? You love to play soccer."

"I'm grown now. I need to work, not play games."

He spun on his heel and ran from the room, tossing his schoolbooks on the table. Miguel heard them slide off and hit the floor but didn't stop. His dreams of a higher education hit the floor with the dead weight of the books. He raced upstairs to his room and slammed the door. His fate had been sealed by a drive-by shooting.

Lupe and Hector sat in the office of their parish priest later that day. Lupe twisted a tissue in her hands shredding the fragile paper. Hector reached over and stilled her fingers, taking her hand in his own.

"Don't worry, we will find out what is troubling our son," he assured her.

"What is worrying you two so much?" Father Enrique asked.

"Our Miguel, Father. He has dropped out of school. He says he doesn't want to go to college. That he is a man and must work to help the family," Lupe cried.

Father Enrique looked concerned. "Do you need his help? Is everything all right at home?"

Hector shook his head. "We don't have lots of money, but we get by. We do not want our children dropping out of school. I learned to be a plumber to pay for them to go to private school so they will get the best education we can afford." He flexed his hands as though to ease aching joints. "It is hard work, but worth every bit of it to give them a better chance than we had. I know that I will have aches and pains later on, and I want better careers for them."

"I thought they had scholarships to the schools?"

"They do, Father. But there are still books to buy, uniforms, fees for sports. But we get by. It is not a problem." He shook his head. "Miguel has no reason to think we must have his help."

"Is there any reason you think he has changed? What else is different?" Father Enrique asked.

Lupe sighed heavily. "He is not my happy Miguel anymore. He is sad and has stopped doing the things he loved. He used to be in the math club and played soccer. He was a star," she said proudly, then she frowned. "For several weeks now, he has been skipping meetings and practices. His coach called and said he hasn't dressed out for soccer in over three weeks. He loved to play sports, but gave it all up today when he dropped out."

"I know one thing that is different. He changed the way he walks to school, and he walks the house at night when he should be sleeping," Hector continued. "He insisted Ruth begin walking Maria to school, too. He refused to do it anymore. We ask him what goes on, but he makes up excuses. He wants more exercise, he claims, so he walks a new way, or he can't sleep. But I know he is having nightmares. I hear him cry out in his sleep."

Father Enrique steepled his fingers, tapping his fore fingers against his chin. Then he dropped his hands to his desk and leaned back in his chair. "Tell Miguel I want him to stay in school until we get this all straightened out. See if you can get him to go back tomorrow and then to come to me after school. We will get to the bottom of this. I'm sure of it."

"Thank you, Father. Bless you," Lupe said, as she slowly got to her feet. The weight of her worry was clear as she turned and left the priest's office.

Miguel slumped in the chair across from Father Enrique. He knew the father meant well, but he had nothing to say to the priest. He couldn't tell anyone what he saw, what he was experiencing. If anyone knew what he experienced that day, and it got back to Alejandro and the gang, he wouldn't see another sunrise. Of that he was sure.

"Miguel, this is our third visit. Don't you know by now you can trust me? Anything you tell me is confidential. You know that."

It was as though the priest could see into his heart, Miguel thought. "No, Father. I mean I don't want to talk. I know I can trust you. I've known you my whole life."

"Miguel, have you done as I asked and gone back to school while we work this out?"

Miguel hung his head for a moment, then lifted his chin and faced the priest eye to eye. "No, Father. I cannot."

"What is it, Miguel? I know you wouldn't drop out willingly. Your teachers say you loved school and always made a contribution in your classes. Something has happened. Why don't you tell me so I can help you?"

"I can't, Father. I am sorry but it is too personal to share." Miguel saw a flicker of curiosity cross Father Enrique's face. What was he thinking? Miguel wondered.

Finally Father Enrique spoke. "Miguel, remember that terrible drive-by shooting at the elementary school?"

Miguel felt the blood drain from his face. Beads of sweat covered his forehead. "Yes."

"Where were you when it happened?"

"School." Miguel looked away, unable to meet Father Enrique's steady gaze.

"What do you remember hearing about it?"

"Not much." He shrugged still looking away.

"Were you afraid for Maria? Isn't that where she goes to school?"

Miguel nodded. "But she was all right when they took them inside and locked it down."

"How do you know that?"

"I saw. . .I mean . . .I knew the teachers would protect her. God would protect her."

Father Enrique sighed. "You saw what happened didn't you, Miguel? Do you know who did this terrible thing?"

Miguel lunged to his feet. "No," he shouted. "I don't know anything. I have to go."

He ran, slamming the door behind him. Miguel left Father Enrique behind and charged down the steps of the church, as though the devil himself were on his heels.

Ethical Points to Consider:

Treating minors involves varying confidentiality and consent issues from state to state. Parents or guardians typically provide consent for the minor to receive treatment. However, laws differ in regard to whether both parents must provide consent and mental health professionals must explore relevant state laws pertaining to non-custodial parents (Remley & Herlihy, 2007). In some states, children and adolescents may be permitted to provide consent for treatment.

Minors, regardless of whether legally providing consent, ethically must be provided with informed consent via a clear explanation in age-appropriate language (ACA, 2005; APA, 2002; NAADAC, 2008; & NASW, 2008). In addition to the typical instances where confidentiality is breached (e.g., imminent harm), minors also need to be aware of information to which their parents/guardians have access. It is critical that the mental health professional be cognizant of relevant laws in his/her state relating to minors and mental health services.

Miguel may reveal who perpetrated the crime during therapy. Assuming Miguel's parents have the right to access information about his counseling and the records, they could find out who committed the crime. The counselor must be careful to inform Miguel, prior to engaging in therapy, what potentially could happen to the information. All aspects of this possibility should be explored with Miguel, prior to beginning counseling.

In the case of Miguel, additional ethical concerns exist regarding competency to provide mental health services. While clergy often have training in pastoral counseling, they recognize the limits of their competency just as ethics codes require mental health workers to (ACA, 2005; APA, 2002; NAADAC, 2008; & NASW, 2008). Father Enrique most likely would refer to a mental health professional because the difficulties Miguel is experiencing are likely beyond his competency. Once Miguel is referred, the possibility of collaboration exists between Father Enrique and the counselor.

Discussion Questions:

1. What are Miguel's important cognitions, emotions, and behaviors? Given your identification of these issues, what theoretical orientation will guide your work with him? How does Miguel's culture impact your conceptualization?

2. Does Miguel fit any diagnostic criteria for a mental disorder? If so, what disorder?

3. How might you collaborate with the priest, Father Enrique, in your work with Miguel? Would you recommend Fr. Enrique do the counseling?

4. Miguel only sees one option to deal with the situation. What options do you see? How will you work with Miguel to have him consider these other options?

5. What cultural factors are relevant to your work with Miguel? If other resources or agencies are involved in this case, what cultural stereotypes about young Latinos might need to be addressed?

6. Family is very important to Miguel. What benefits and drawbacks are there to including Miguel's family in treatment? Are there pre-existing family issues that might impact treatment? Commitment to treatment can be a significant issue in family therapy. How would you address this?

7. Assume while in therapy, Miguel discloses who perpetrated the crime. How would you balance Miguel's rights to confidentiality, the rights of his parents to information and the possibility of them informing the police, with Miguel's fears for his safety?

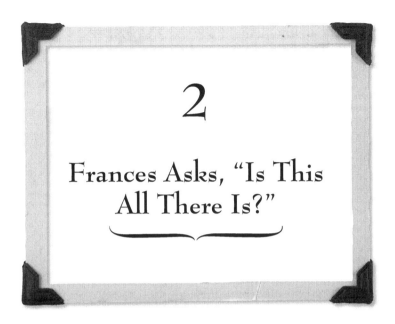

2

Frances Asks, "Is This All There Is?"

For Your Consideration

As you read the following case, think about possible short- and long-term goals you would have when counseling Frances. Consider stereotyped role expectations and their impact.

Frances's Story

Frances slid behind the wheel of her BMW, slammed the car door, and reviewed the list she pulled from her purse. A glance in the rearview mirror assured her she had picked up the dry cleaning, now hanging inside the back door. The mirror reflected the fresh, platinum blond highlights Ted liked her to keep. Her face had been treated, plucked and polished. God, she hated beauty parlor days. What a waste of time, she thought. All in the name of being the beautiful trophy wife at Ted's client parties.

"Do your part," she muttered. "Ted does the hard work. All you have to do is entertain his guests." She scoffed at that idea, when a picture of her Swedish immigrant father working their Imperial Valley farm year round to keep them going popped into her head. Ted's job might be stressful, but it didn't have anything to do with hard physical labor. The large agri-businesses had finally taken her father's farm over, and instead of being able to retire in peace, he'd died of a broken heart at eighty.

Frances thought again of the soft work Ted did as an advertising executive and of the part she played. She shuddered. Could she stand one more boring party, talking about things she had no interest in or, worse yet, listening to the wives gossip about what went on in the company? Some days she just wanted the world to stop so she could leap off. The thought brought a smile to her lips. She could imagine Ted's chagrin if she disappeared when he needed her the most, to keep someone's wife out of the way, while he made a business deal with the woman's husband. It might just be worth it, she thought.

"Get real, girl. Where would you go?" she asked the empty car. Moving down the list, she checked off the stops she'd made. Grocery bags filled the trunk and the bank statement sat on the seat beside her. Frances's stomach grumbled. It was nearly lunchtime. She still needed to put all this stuff away and clean up the house, before Ted got home from work.

Grabbing her cell phone, Frances hit auto dial for the pizza place. She ordered a pizza with everything, even anchovies, and knew she'd get to the house in time for it to be delivered. Frances deserved a treat after a morning of torture at the salon, didn't she? Ted would never know. She put the car in gear, backed out and headed for home. Something is really wrong with me if I get this much enjoyment out of something as simple as sidestepping Ted's control over my diet, she thought.

Later that afternoon, inside their beautifully decorated Tudor house, Frances fanned the sweat from her face, once again cursing menopause. At fifty-nine, she had hoped she was mostly past that phase of her life, but it seemed to be hanging on. In her former life as a nun, she was made to believe in a punishing God.

"Perhaps this is His idea of retribution," she grumbled. As it always seemed to when she was reminded of menopause and her less than perfect body, Frances's mood slipped into the dark.

Frances glanced at the kitchen clock while she dried her hands on a tea towel and gasped when she realized how late it was. Ted would be home any minute. She pushed away from the counter, threw the towel down, and hurried across to the breakfast nook. She scooped up the now empty pizza box.

As Frances opened the lid to confirm she had, in fact, eaten the entire extra large pizza alone, a tear slipped from her eye and trailed down her cheek, as guilt hit her right between the eyes. She sniffed the air and realized it still smelled of tomato sauce, several meat toppings, veggies, anchovies, and cheese. It couldn't get much more telltale than that, she thought. Frances grabbed a can of vanilla air freshener out from under the sink and blasted the kitchen with it, then lit a couple of scented candles to help cover the pizza odor. Ted would have plenty to say if he saw what she'd done — again. It was getting more difficult to hide the evidence every couple days. Not that she didn't give herself enough grief over her binge eating, she thought. He didn't have to remind her she'd gained twenty-three pounds during her fifties. She would fast the next couple of days to offset the pizza. She knew it without anyone reminding her about it. She scowled. Why couldn't people just mind their own business? Frances was really tired of trying to live up to others' expectations for her. According to Ted and her mother, it mattered what other people thought of her. Frances was finding it difficult to care anymore what anyone thought, even her family.

The thought took her back 50 years to the first time she tried to tell her mother about her uncle abusing her. Teresa had been furious. How dare Frances say such a vile thing? No one in their family would commit such a horrible act. Keep your wild, lustful fantasies to yourself, she'd screamed at Frances. Mind your business and don't speak to anyone of such false tales. Who did she think she was to accuse a fine man like Uncle Lars? People would say Frances had led him on and seduced him with her wicked ways, her mother had said. She was to never tell a soul about these allegations — ever.

Frances had known she should show her mother the physical proof, the bites on her small breasts, the bruising in her pubic area; she couldn't. She was too ashamed. Frances had felt filthy and unworthy then. Maybe her mother was right. Maybe she had led him on somehow, been responsible for what happened to her. Maybe she was being punished for something she didn't understand.

She still bore the scars from years of abuse, both physical and emotional. Maybe Daddy would have helped, she thought, but no. She couldn't do that. She couldn't go to him. He'd stop loving her if he knew what she did with Uncle Lars. It was an evil thing, and she had played a part in it. No, Daddy was the only one who loved her, so she couldn't risk that.

"Mind your own business. Keep it to yourself," Mother said. So that's what she'd do, she'd thought then. After that first time of seeking help from her mother to make it stop, she never mentioned it again. What was the point? She was on her own.

Frances shook her head to clear the cobwebs of the past and drew her attention back to the box in her hands. *Nothing is anybody else's business and that includes what I choose to eat.*

She crammed the box into a huge, dark trash bag, and then scurried around the house picking up trash from the other rooms before closing the bag and placing it outside in the garbage can. She dusted her hands after sealing the lid, knowing Ted wouldn't go near the trash and no one would know what she'd done — this time. Except of course when her weight shot up a few pounds, Ted always noticed that.

Her shoulders sagged as she dragged her over-stuffed body back into the kitchen through the garage. Frances shook her head as she thought of the headache and lethargy that would follow eating the junk food. Her depression would deepen, too. It always did after a binge. Why couldn't she stop eating when she knew how badly it affected her body and her weight?

Frances sniffed at the air. The freshener had worked. Her gaze slid across the spotless room. Not a thing out of place, not a speck of dust, a crumb or a dirty dish. She cleaned constantly to occupy the empty, daytime hours since her last child had moved away to college. She felt she had nothing to fill her time, although Ted insisted she play bridge and go to bingo games. A disgusted sigh slipped through her lips at the thought of one more boring, inane afternoon of bingo or bridge.

"He's trying to help you," she chastised out loud. But the games had long since lost their fun factor, and she dreaded spending time with other women with no more to discuss than pregnant daughters, potty training grandbabies, and the upcoming church yard sale. She'd tried interjecting some current events, talked a bit about art and history. The others had looked at her like she'd lost her mind. It was apparent they wondered why she'd care about any of those other topics. Their lives revolved around their families. Why isn't that enough for me anymore? she wondered. Frances loved all of her children and took great pride in their success. When they left, my life ended, she thought.

"You're getting morbid," she scolded. Hmmm . . . maybe a call to Cynthia will help, she thought. It had been months since she'd seen her best friend for lunch. Cynthia was always so busy. A high level manager for a national disaster relief group, it seemed she was constantly on the run with meetings, fund raising, and travel.

Frances walked to the kitchen desk and stared at the phone. She started to pick it up, and then dropped her hand, moving over to get a glass of water from the sink. She moved back to the phone and swung away one more time. She felt wired. Restless. What the devil's the matter with you? Settle down and call Cynthia, she told herself. Frances finally snatched up the phone and dialed before she could change her mind. She quickly learned from Cynthia's administrative assistant she was out of the office and could be reached on her cell phone. Frances tried that number and Cynthia answered on the second ring.

"Hi, Cynthia, how are you?"

"Packing. What are you up to?" Her voice sounded distracted.

"Nothing, as usual. Where you headed?"

"Alabama."

The short answers told Frances what she needed to know. Cynthia was headed out again and she needed to hurry. No time for old friends today.

"What's up down there?"

"Massive streak of tornados. They need our help."

Frances could hear Cynthia opening and closing drawers, then the sound of a suitcase zipper.

"Sorry, Franny. I have to run. The plane to Montgomery is in two hours. Once I have everything set there, they are sending me overseas to check on some of our foreign units helping in Indonesia. Call you when I get back and we'll get together."

"Have a safe —" The phone went dead in her hand before she could finish. Frances stared at the receiver willing her friend's voice back, but it didn't work.

She slowly replaced it and sighed. Cynthia had important work to do. People depended on her. Frances knew from past experience that Cynthia could organize anything, including millions of dollars worth of supplies and assistance to those in dire straits, and she could do it fast. What could I do? she wondered. Could she work for some important organization? Frances scoffed at the idea. No one would want an old, former convent nurse turned stay-at-home mom.

Listlessly, she trailed her fingers over the counter before stopping at the cabinet with her pills. Frances lifted a hand to open the door, dropped it again, and then with a sigh, gave up and opened the cabinet. She took one bottle down and stared at the label. Ted hated it when she relied on pills. Her shoulders drooped as though the weight of the world rested on them. Maybe she just needed a change, something to shake things up, she thought. Oh well, like that's going to happen. The pills helped some, but lately, something was missing and the hole in her heart was growing bigger and deeper every day.

Her days were taken up with filling other people's needs. Hadn't she always done that as a child, she thought. Bile rose in her throat as she thought of her uncle, molesting her fragile young body, of her mother who denied the truth rather than face it. Spending her childhood in hiding and working around home nonstop instead of being cared for.

She shook her head. What had she chosen for work — nursing. She was still caring for everyone else. Frances smiled to herself. She had loved the religious life at the convent. Her smile faded. Controversy had become hostile by the late '60s. The issue of women's equality became a big problem in the church, a problem that really concerned her until finally it was bad enough she had left. And of course, after that, she spent her life caring for Ted and their children. It seemed she had always been a mother in one way or another.

The electronic garage door opened, and she heard the sound of Ted's Mercedes pulling in. Frances hurriedly put the pill bottle back on the shelf and slammed the cabinet door. She moved to the sink, grabbed a glass and filled it with cool water. She was drinking it when Ted came in.

He walked in loosening his tie and slapped his briefcase down on the kitchen counter. "Hi, Hon." He bussed her cheek with an absent-minded kiss. "How are you?"

Frances tried to smile but knew it didn't reach her eyes. "All right, I guess. How —?"

"Man, what a day." He walked to the liquor cabinet and made himself a gin and tonic without offering Frances anything. "I had to meet with a bunch of new out-of-town clients at the Plaza for lunch. After that they insisted on going to the museum of art history, before we went back to the meeting in the boardroom." He turned his back on her and moved toward the living room.

"Ted, let's go out —"

"That Sanderson hogged the whole show talking to the clients in Japanese, while I sat there like a fool." He dropped down in his recliner, not even bothering to go and change to casual clothes first.

Tears welled in Frances's eyes. "Ted, I'm trying to ask you something."

He looked startled as though he hadn't even heard her speak. "Sorry, Babe. What is it? Bad day at the bridge club?"

His sarcasm bit into her. "You're the one who wants me to play." She took a deep breath. "No, it has nothing to do with that. I just want to get out of here for a while. Let's go out for dinner. Someplace new and . . . and different. I heard about a great new Thai restaurant across town."

Ted groaned. "Frances, I'm beat tonight. Can't it wait? I really just want to stay home. As soon as I drink this," he lifted the glass, "I'm going to change into jeans and kick back. It's been a long day."

"You think it wasn't a long day for me? Running errands all morning. Nothing exciting to do? I'm tired of not doing anything but taking care of this house and taking care of you. I need something. . . more, Ted."

"You go to the club. You have your friends. What more do you need? I work my ass off to give you everything, to keep this big house. I'm tired. Don't be selfish, Frances. I want to stay home tonight." He snatched up the newspaper she had left beside his chair and flipped it open to the financial page. From behind the paper he said, "Besides we have the black tie fund raiser Saturday night at the club. You can wait until then, can't you? Wear that great red dress, why don't you? It'll make you feel better."

Frances spun on her heel and hurried to the bedroom, slamming the door behind her. "Don't be selfish." She had heard the words repeated time and again in her youth. If it wasn't from her mother, it was from the culture in which she was raised. Mothers had to serve, to care for others without regard for themselves. So she'd slaved, and worked, and raised her children to be successful. And where were they now? They were all gone, she was alone, and had nothing left but the duty of seeing to her aged mother's needs, once in a while, when her brother couldn't. Of course, that meant risking running into Uncle Lars. Oh, she still took care of her husband, but when would she ever have the right to take care of herself? she wondered. And even if she could, what the devil did she want? What was missing that seemed to leave such a huge hole in her life?

Leaning against the closed door, she let her gaze slide around the perfectly decorated and made-up room. Dinner dance on Saturday night. Guess she'd have to look forward to that. The thought of spending several hours with a bunch of stuffed shirts, who only new how to talk financials, made her groan. "Right, and I enjoy the dentist, too."

She pushed away from the door and went to her closet. The fire red dress that was Ted's favorite hung there. Frances thought about pushing it aside, out of spite. "Don't be selfish." Her shoulders sagged, and she took the dress out to try it on. It had been six months since she'd had an occasion to wear it.

Stripped down to her underwear, she pulled the dress over her head. She fought to slide the tight skirt over her hips. When she had it pulled down, she turned to see the back zipper. A good two inches separated the fabric sides. There was no way she could fit into this dress and wear it in public. A sob escaped as her mood sank more.

Tears streamed down Frances's face as she fought her way out of the tight dress, tugging and jerking it until she feared it would rip apart at the seams. She'd never been good enough. Not for Ted, the children, her mother. Only her father had loved her unconditionally, she thought.

Only he thought she could have done more, been more, experienced more. But it was too late now, wasn't it? Maybe she should give up the worldly things and go back to the convent. She could hide there. She shook her head as she swiped the moisture from her cheeks. Frances knew that wasn't what she was seeking either. Women were no more equal there than in this house. Was keeping house and working at a less than satisfying marriage all she had to look forward to? Is this all there is to life? she wondered. She'd watched her father die, her mother fade, her husband and children succeed. Her entire life, Frances had only accepted the leftovers of time, money, even love. Nothing had been freely given to her; many things had been forced on her.

The sound of Ted coming down the hall made her throw the dress down in a heap of red satin. She bolted for the master bath, closing the door so he couldn't see her ravaged face.

"Hey, Hon. Where'd you go? Aren't we going to eat?"

"Later. I'll fix something later." Her voice made a strangled sound, forced from her tightened throat. She didn't really care if he heard.

As silent sobs filled her chest and overflowed, she thought of her father and her beloved brother, Peter, who had died in Viet Nam. Maybe she would find peace if she went to be with them. Frances thought briefly of suicide once again. She'd missed her brother and father terribly, longed to see them again, and perhaps find the peace she believed they knew now. Frances shook the thoughts away.

"Keep it together, girl. Suicide is not an option," she said to herself. "What would my kids do if I wasn't here for them?" A soul-deep sigh filled the bathroom. "It's hopeless. I am hopeless."

As sobs shook her shoulders, she slid down the bathroom door and covered her face with her hands. Frances realized it was time to get professional help. She needed to find some answers and prayed someone could help her find them.

Ethical Points to Consider:

This case presents interesting ethical scenarios. Mandatory child abuse reporting exists nationwide for numerous professions. Ethical codes require informing clients prior to treatment of confidentiality exceptions such as mandated reporting (ACA, 2005; APA, 2002; NAADAC, 2008; & NASW, 2008). In this case however, the victim is no longer a child and the perpetrator is elderly. State laws vary in addressing this circumstance.

Initially, the counselor must consider whether the abuser has access to victims and whether perpetration is continuing. Additionally, are there any identifiable victims to warn? Remley and Herlihy (2007) point out the importance of checking mandatory reporting laws in regard to previous abuse. Further, Remley and Herlihy caution that reports that are not legally mandated may result in the counselor being unprotected in relation to making the report.

This case points out the importance of working closely with child protection agencies. An information-only call would clarify laws which apply to reporting when the abuse is in the distant past. Establishing contacts that include lawyers and caseworkers cannot be overemphasized. Their expertise can prove invaluable. However, it remains critical for the mental health worker to review applicable laws for the situation and extensively document the information, therapist's actions, and decisions.

A suicide assessment needs to be done with Frances. Bennett, Bricklin, Harris, Knapp, VandeCreek, and Younggren (2006), suggest suicide assessments include: predisposition, impulsiveness, previous behaviors, hopelessness, symptoms, stressors, suicide plan, intensity of the thoughts, frequency of thoughts, symptoms, support systems, and coping strategies. Depending on the dangerousness, a suicide safety contract might be developed. Clients at high risk often need hospitalization. Knowledge of ethical codes and state laws regarding involuntary hospitalization and duty to warn guide counselors in this area.

Discussion Questions:

1. What are Frances's key cognitions, emotions, and behaviors that you will integrate into your counseling? Given your identification of these issues, what theoretical orientation would you choose in your work with her? How do you conceptualize the case? What specific techniques and treatment plan would you employ?

2. Does Frances meet the criteria for a diagnosis? If so, which diagnosis(es)?

3. How has her cultural background shaped her cognitive and behavioral choices?

4. How might Frances's former life as a nun affect her current behavioral choices?

5. What purpose does food serve for Frances?

6. How do society's messages about appropriate roles for women and men affect Frances's life? How will they affect your work with her — and her husband if you see him in counseling? How might your own views about gender roles affect your work with her?

7. How does the past child sexual abuse and her mother's response to her disclosure affect Frances's current self-concept?

8. Are there ethical or legal mandated reporting requirements?

9. What is her current potential for suicide? What are the factors that make it more likely? Less likely?

10. What strengths or assets does Frances have that you will build on in your counseling?

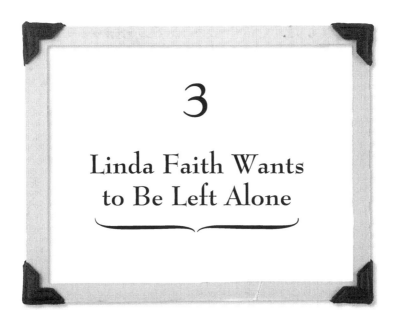

3

Linda Faith Wants to Be Left Alone

For Your Consideration

As you read the following case, be aware of your biases toward different treatment modalities and reactions toward the characters. How do
your perspectives impact your opinions regarding removing Linda Faith
from her family to focus on herself versus having the family enter family
therapy or couples therapy? What cultural expectations and pressures are
influencing Linda Faith and her family?

Linda Faith's Story

Linda Faith landed on the mat with perfect form. Her coach called
out, "Way to go" and her teammates clapped. Linda Faith pulled at
the bottom of her royal blue leotard, tugging it down over thin hips. The
fabric did little to hide her pointed hipbones. She shook her head as she
walked to Mr. Dunagan.

"That wasn't good, Coach," she said as he handed her a sweat towel.

"It was excellent, Linda Faith." He grasped her shoulders and gave them a gentle squeeze. "You are doing great this year and will make it onto the Junior Varsity team next fall."

She shook her head, dropping her chin onto her chest. "I'm not good enough for them."

He lifted her chin so she had to look at him. "I'm the coach, you're the gymnast. I say you're good enough." His gaze slid over her, and she fought the urge to squirm. "I am worried though, Linda Faith."

She ran a hand over her slim waist to her hipbone. She looked down at herself. "Am I still too heavy. I can lose some more weight, limber up more."

"No. You're a little *too* thin. I don't want you to lose any more weight. Stay just like you are or add a couple of pounds."

She looked at him, tried to assess whether he was being honest or not. "Don't lose any more weight?"

"No, you're fine. And give yourself a break. That was a great parallel bar routine. Go get cleaned up."

"Yes, Coach." She turned away but not before she caught a glimpse of herself in the workout mirrors along the wall. She stopped for a second, pinched a tiny bit of skin together, and decided she was still too fat. She'd have to fix that, she thought, and hurried to change into jogging clothes. Linda Faith still had time to get a couple of miles in, before her mother came for her.

Michelle St. Clair watched her daughter walk toward the car an hour later. She smiled at her daughter's perfection: blond hair, blue eyes, slim, athletic . . . everything she'd wanted in a daughter. Sarah Grace was nearly perfect, but heavier. Her younger daughter could stand to lose ten pounds.

Linda Faith threw her gym bag in the back and climbed in on the passenger side. "Hi, Mom."

"Hi, Sweetie. How was the practice?"

She shrugged. "Okay, I guess. Coach said it was good."

"And what did you think of your performance?"

Linda Faith made a face. "I think I need to spend a few hours at the gym Saturday to get in some more practice before the meet next week."

Michelle nodded. "That can be arranged."

"Thanks. Can we go home now? I want to practice my piano lessons before Dad and Sarah Grace get home."

"All right. I'll drop you off and then run to the store. What do you want for dinner?"

"Not much. Something fat free would be good." She shrugged. "I don't care what, as long as it's healthy."

Michelle slid her gaze over her daughter's figure. It's great she is slim, but she needs to start developing — a figure — hell even start her menstrual cycle — anything at all, so she starts growing up. If not, how is she ever going to get into my sorority and find a nice boy to marry? Her husband, David, insisted Linda Faith was losing too much weight and needed to eat like a normal teenager. Michelle huffed out a breath. Like either of their daughters was merely normal. Who knew better about what their children needed than their mother? Certainly not the father.

"What's Sarah Grace doing tonight?" Linda Faith asked.

"She's over at the community center. That boy she likes ... um ...."

"Joe," Linda Faith supplied.

Michelle frowned. "Yes, Joe, he talked her into volunteering to work with some of the younger kids on their little stage play for the Spring Fling."

"Better her than me." Linda Faith shuddered. "I wouldn't want to have anything to do with drama."

"You know, your gymnastics and diving takes you in front of people. This is not much different."

"I don't have to say anything. All I have to do is what I like."

"What about the piano? You don't like to play it when anyone is home. How will you do a recital?"

"I won't," she said firmly. "I play for myself." She stared out the window avoiding her mother's gaze as they pulled into the driveway of their upscale Atlanta home.

Michelle stopped trying to talk to Linda Faith and gazed at the antebellum house on the hill. The drive wound through landscaped lawns, peach trees heavy with blossoms, and flowerbeds bursting with color. Their gardeners did an amazing job on it she had to admit. And whether she resented his time away as an attorney or not, David did provide for his family's every want and need. She resented that he seemed to have forgotten the part she played in his success. With a degree in business, she had worked to put him through Stanford. When times were really tough, it had been her parents who had kept them afloat.

Suppressed anger fought with the gratitude she felt for all David gave her and the girls. She may be grateful to have met and married him, to have had two beautiful daughters, but she'd never forgive him for the affair he'd had last summer. Oh, he'd been full of apologies and seemed truly penitent at the time, but Michelle suspected it wasn't the first, or the last time, he'd strayed from home.

The car pulled up in front of the house and Linda Faith jumped out, grabbing her bag from the rear seat. "See you later, Mom."

"I won't be long. Have a good piano practice."

Michelle watched Linda Faith go in the front door before pulling away. She wondered what she could get her daughter to eat that might help her stop losing weight. She knew David would have a fit if his daughter didn't eat a decent meal soon.

Linda Faith pushed the food around her plate, barely touching a thing. Michelle glanced nervously from her to David and back. She knew David was watching Linda Faith to see how well she ate.

Michelle pushed a bowl of vegetables toward her daughter. "Here, Dear, have some more. These are good for you."

"No thanks, Mom. I'm not hungry. I had a protein shake while I practiced piano. May I be excused?"

"No!"

"Sure." Michelle spoke at the same time as David. She saw the glance that Linda Faith sent between them and simply nodded at her daughter, allowing her to escape the coming explosion.

"You have got to stop allowing her to eat like that," David snapped. "She's losing too much weight."

Michelle got up and carried plates to the sink, scraping Linda Faith's food into the garbage disposal. "She's fine. Stop worrying."

"One of us has to." David pushed his chair back from the table so hard it toppled behind him. "You don't give a damn about her unless she fits your ideal."

"That's not true." She stopped what she was doing and picked up a dishtowel to dry her hands. Slowly she turned toward David. "I only want what she does."

"Oh, I guess if all she wanted was sex or drugs you'd let her do that, too."

"Don't be ridiculous," Michelle ground out.

"I'm not. This eating problem is getting out of hand, and it is as destructive to her as the other things. We've got to do something."

"She knows her own body. She says she's fine."

"You want it to be fine so she can compete," he shouted. He threw down the cloth napkin in his hand. "You don't give a damn about her, only your own lost dreams of competing."

Michelle felt the blood drain from her face and reached behind her to hold on to the counter top. "You son-of-a-bitch, nothing I've ever done has been good enough for you. That's why you went outside our marriage for your sex games."

"Oh, for Pete's sake. Are you ever going to stop throwing that in my face? I said I was sorry. You live in this fine house, eat good food, drink fine wine. I don't see you complaining about any of that." He was no longer shouting, but Michelle heard the upstairs bathroom door slam and knew Linda Faith had listened to all of it from the landing.

"Never mind," she said, suddenly tired. "I don't want to talk about this. I'll talk to her coach and see what he says, then I'll do what I can to get her to stop losing weight." She took a deep breath and slowly let it out. "Good enough?"

"It will have to be. If anything happens to her, it will be your fault for letting this continue. Put your foot down for once and tell her to sit down at the table and stay there until she eats a decent meal."

"I don't think it will work, but I'll try. I'll check into some other options for her as well, but I still say she is just going through a phase.

She desperately wants to win this meet and to be picked up for the high school varsity team."

Michelle thought of her daughter's request to work out for several hours on Saturday, and she wondered what David would have to say about the extra physical activity.

"Will you be home this weekend?" she asked.

She watched his gaze slide over her, wondered if he'd ever again look at her like he had in the early days of their marriage.

"No, I don't think so. I've got a big case coming up. I'll be at my office all day Saturday, maybe even Sunday."

"Fine. I'll take care of things, just like always."

She spun on her heel and left the kitchen, leaving him standing at the table.

Two weeks later, she watched Linda Faith compete and win the meet, get chosen for the high school team, and get promoted from sophomore to junior. Time was flying by, and her two daughters would soon be graduating high school.

August rolled around and Michelle wondered why Linda Faith had given up swimming in the family pool. Whenever she saw her, she had on a winter jogging outfit of velour in her trademark royal blue. It was only 8 a.m. when she saw her jog up the long winding driveway.

Michelle straightened up and pulled off her gardening gloves. The gardeners weren't crazy about her getting into the beds, but she enjoyed transplanting flowers and being outside, especially when David was inside.

She waved at Linda Faith and called her over. "Aren't you hot in that, dear? The humidity is evil this morning." She looked at the sweat pouring off her daughter's face. Her face seemed swollen. Hipbones protruded through the velour. Had they been like that a month ago, even a week ago?

"I'm fine, Mom. I'll just go shower."

"Why don't you take a dip in the pool and cool off? You have an extra suit in the pool house."

"Oh, I don't think so. Since Dad's leaving for work and Sarah Grace is at the community center, I want to practice piano. I'll just go in."

She turned away from Michelle and walked toward the house. One leg of her jogging pants pulled up a bit, and Michelle nearly gasped when she saw the lower part of Linda Faith's leg. She knew she could easily wrap her thumb and forefinger around the entire thing and would come close to touching her fingers together. She let her gaze go up Linda Faith's back and saw shoulder blades pressed against the fabric.

David had been right. Their daughter was starving to death before their very eyes. Michelle dropped her gloves in the grass, and hurried inside to call the in-patient program the school nurse had told her about in May. They couldn't wait any longer to let Linda Faith correct the situation herself.

"Linda Faith, I'm Roger. Have a seat." He looked at the small blonde sitting across from him. She looked much younger than her actual fourteen years. A strong wind would blow you away, he thought.

The girl kept her eyes downcast, and on the rare occasion she looked up, she glared at him. The parents were on either side of her, seeming to trap her and give her no escape route.

"I know you don't want to be here, but you've got a problem Linda."

"Linda Faith," the mother said. "And this," she indicated another daughter sitting on the loveseat to the side, "is Sarah Grace."

"Excuse me," Roger said. "Linda Faith, you have a problem and we can't help you if you don't let us. The whole family came with you today to do the intake. You'll be with us for several months."

Linda Faith bolted to her feet. "I can't! School starts in two weeks. I can't stay here. I have to compete on the team."

David caught her arm and gently pulled her down. "Sit down. Listen to what he has to say."

"You will continue your schoolwork here while you participate in counseling and group sessions," Roger continued. His voice was deliberately calm, trying to ease the energy he felt pulsing from Linda Faith and her family. There was no doubt the girl had been living in chaos for some time. Roger had spoken to her teachers and learned she was only receiving B's and C's, but they felt she was quite smart, perhaps even gifted.

"Linda Faith, your teachers tell me you do really well in school. Do you like it?"

She shrugged, refusing to speak.

"What about your friends? Do you have a best friend or two?"

Linda Faith shook her head, all the while keeping her chin dropped onto her chest and not meeting his eyes.

"Young lady, answer Mr. Hansen's questions," her father snapped.

"That's all right. We'll get to know each other in the coming days." Roger closed the file on his desk and got to his feet. "Girls, will you excuse us for a few minutes? I want to speak to your parents."

The two sisters stood, eyed the counselor somewhat suspiciously, and then slipped from the room.

"What else can we do to help?" Michelle asked.

Roger sat down and re-opened the file. "Can you tell me how your family life has been the last two years or so? Are you having problems at home?"

"I don't see where our marriage has anything to do with Linda Faith's problems." David frowned and picked imaginary lint off his trousers, obviously reluctant to speak about this aspect of their lives.

"I didn't specifically mention your marriage, but we can talk about that, too, since it sounds like there may be some problems. You can help me help Linda Faith by being open about anything disturbing that has been happening at home. I can help her by getting to know these relationships within the family." He was silent for a moment as the discomfort in the room escalated. "If we help Linda Faith with her disorder and send her home to the same situation she's in now, she will very likely suffer a relapse. If she does, she can do permanent damage to her body. Deadly damage." He let the last fall on the quiet parents.

Michelle gasped and David visibly struggled to maintain his composure. At last the husband spoke. "What do you need to know?"

"Good. Now we can start in earnest. Let me call the girls back in."

When they were seated Roger continued the intake. "Tell me about the family over the last two years. What's different in life for you, Linda Faith?"

"Nothing, everything is perfect except for this. I finally am reaching my dream of being a gymnast. I work hard at school and practice my piano. Just when everything is almost perfect, you all conspire to screw me." She nearly screamed it. "I'm missing gymnastics, piano, school, and everything I need to get done. I refuse to let you keep me here."

"Me, me, me! I'm missing things at the community center that are important, just to be here and hear more about you." Sarah Grace yelled back.

"Girls, this is not how ladies act," Michelle said.

"Sarah Grace, how do you see Linda Faith? You sound angry," Roger commented.

"She has her life and I have mine. I love her but we do different things. If she decides to starve to death, it is her right. I didn't cause it. I have events planned at the community center. Joe and I have plans later."

"Don't you want to help her?" Roger watched the girl, saw her gaze slide over her sister, then come back to him.

"This is ridiculous. It has nothing to do with me. I am doing what I am supposed to and being made to suffer all because of her. Keep her, let her go — whatever. I am so sick of hearing day and night about Linda Faith and food. You think you refuse to do this," she said glaring at Linda Faith, "well so do I. Joe will come pick me up. Later." Sarah Grace jumped to her feet and stormed out of the room.

Roger looked at the surprised faces of the family and asked, "Does her leaving concern anyone?" When the three of them just shrugged their shoulders, Roger went on with the intake session. "Linda Faith, tell me how you lost the 40 pounds?"

"Everyone knows that being a gymnast requires a perfect body. I needed to get in shape. I refuse to stay here and have you ruin what I have worked so hard for."

David, who had been quiet through most of the session finally stood and indicated Michelle should do likewise. He looked down on his daughter and with surrender evident in his voice, said, "You don't have a choice, Linda Faith, and neither do we. We're leaving and you're staying. We'll be back when Mr. Hansen tells us we can visit."

With Michelle clinging to his arm, they quietly left the office, leaving Linda Faith behind pleading with Roger to set her free.

Ethical Points to Consider:

This case centers on the right to refuse treatment. State laws mandate the age of consent for treatment, conversely the age at which one can refuse treatment when involuntary commitment is not involved. We know Linda Faith is starting her junior year in high school from the introduction and can assume she is 15 or 16. Depending on the state, she is old enough to consent to treatment.

Ethical codes dictate that when clients are minors, counselors work to gain their consent to treatment and minimally that the client understands treatment (ACA, 2005; & NASW, 2008). The counselor must balance Linda Faith's refusing treatment with her parents wanting her in counseling. Given her situation, the counselor believes she needs treatment. Overall, clients are more amenable to treatment when they select it, versus being forced or mandated. The counselor in this case would be well advised to work with Linda Faith, so that she sees the potential benefits of treatment. Although, her parents might legally force her (as a minor) into treatment, it is important that Linda Faith be agreeable. Clearly, there is denial of the problem by Linda Faith. Treatment will address her denial, however, if she does not become amenable to treatment and continually fights it or fakes her way through it, she is not likely to experience the short- or long-term benefits of therapy.

Discussion Questions:

1. What cognitions, emotions and behaviors are apparent in Linda Faith and her family? Given these would you recommend treatment? For who and with what theoretical orientation? Describe how you would conceptualize this case and envision treatment progressing.

2. Does Linda Faith meet the criteria for a diagnosis? If so, with what disorder(s)? What disorders, if any, do her family members have?

3. How do societal and cultural forces impact this case?

4. How might inpatient treatment be beneficial in some ways and not others for Linda Faith?

5. What, if any, adjuncts to therapy would you recommend and for what purpose?

6. Would you require couples and/or family therapy as a part of treatment? Justify your decision.

7. How would you address Linda Faith's refusing treatment?

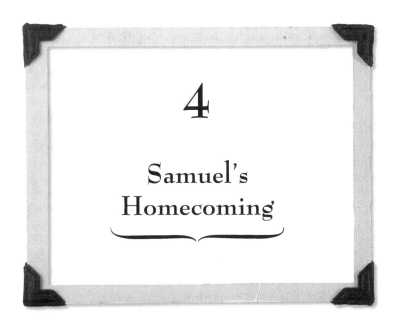

4

Samuel's Homecoming

For Your Consideration

As you read the following case, be aware of the various cultures involved and how the cultures collide. Each of us has political viewpoints and thoughts about war, how do yours influence you? How do your cognitive and emotional reactions impact your empathy and reactions to the situation? How do economic and cultural factors impact this case?

Samuel's Story

Samuel thrust another pan of chicken fried steak into the warming table, so his crew could serve the soldiers coming through the line. They had to eat fast and get back on duty. Samuel watched the men and women around the tables wolfing down food, silent, thinking. He wondered if they thought this might be their last meal. There isn't any way to relax here, he thought.

From the distance came the rumble of an explosion. Samuel knew his Navajo parents had hoped he'd be farther back from the front lines. His mother, Wanda, was a weaver and his father, John, a construction worker on the reservation. He'd hoped Samuel would follow his footsteps after high school, but Sam discovered he enjoyed cooking instead. Besides, this was where he was needed. The soldiers up here had to eat, too, and if he could cook nourishing meals for them, that was his contribution to this war. At least he could tell his mother he wasn't a foot soldier, dodging bullets, mines, and car bombs.

The enemy was everywhere. You couldn't tell who was a good guy and who was a terrorist in this country. From the deserts of New Mexico and Arizona, he knew sand when he saw it, but this country was unbelievably hot, dry, and sandy compared to the U.S. deserts. At home, to the west he had plateaus, some high mountains, running creeks, and cedar and piñon trees with hot, sandy, flatter lands to the east.

"Hey, Sam, get a move on, will ya?"

He jumped and cleared his head of the images. There wasn't time to daydream. He had work to do. "Yes, Master Sergeant. Right away."

He hurried to the back, grabbed another pan of food and brought it out, then went back to his stove to keep cooking. It was a constant job to keep the rotating soldiers fed. He did the best he could in the circumstances, with canned goods and food they were sent to prepare. It was better than the rations they got during maneuvers, but not by much.

His maternal great-grandfather, Running Deer, had been a Navajo code talker during WWII. The day after Pearl Harbor, Running Deer had enlisted, just as Samuel enlisted right after 9/11. He had done his best to take care of the soldiers he was with by sending messages in Navajo so the enemy couldn't break the code. Samuel was determined to care for his soldiers, too, and, even though not an officer, he considered these soldiers he fed as his.

Most of the supplies he cooked with were shipped in, but to try to liven things up a bit, he was sent by his sergeant into the local markets so he could buy what was fresh. He glanced around the tent kitchen and realized supplies were getting pretty well depleted. He decided that after lunch was done, he'd hurry into the town and get some fresh food.

When the last soldier cleared the serving area, Samuel put his crew in charge of cleanup and pulled off his apron. Snatching up his hat, he called out to the soldiers parked in front of the tent.

"Hey, can I have a ride into town? I want to pick up some supplies."

"Sure, come on," the Sergeant said. "Hurry it up, though, we have to get moving."

Samuel hurried to the vehicle and jumped into the open back. They headed down the shell-pitted dirt path, dodging holes and piles of debris. His gaze slid across the barren landscape, over bombed out buildings, and sad-eyed children.

In town, they quickly handled their business, going their own ways and meeting up again an hour later. When they returned for him, Samuel piled his goods in the back of the vehicle, turning to get one last load from the sidewalk.

An explosion tore through the air, sending Samuel flying ten feet up before slamming him against a building. He crumpled on the dirt beside it. He felt his ribs shatter from the hit and instinctively reached to protect them. Blood poured from his severely damaged right hand.

The screams and curses of the others jerked him back to the moment. With adrenaline rushing through his body, he jumped to his feet and raced for the vehicle where his buddies were trapped. Smoke poured from under the vehicle's hood. It would be only a matter of seconds before the whole thing blew. One by one he pulled the seriously wounded men from the vehicle, only to drop them in the dirt and race back for another until all five were clear of the burning wreck. When they were all out, Samuel slumped to the ground holding his ribs with his bleeding hand, and prayed for medical help soon, or they would all die.

Things happened fast when help finally arrived. The men were triaged, and loaded up in order of the severity of their wounds. Samuel refused to be taken away until all the others were put into U.S. vehicles and headed for help. He knew without being told, they were all going home now. There wasn't any more they could do here in the shape they were in. Their tours were over.

At the military hospital stateside, Samuel slowly recovered physically. His ribs healed, and his hand began to mend. He knew he had a long road ahead of him: surgeries, physical therapy, and a lot of painkillers. Within two weeks, he'd been discharged from the Army and transferred to a veteran's hospital for recovery.

A soft tap on the door drew his attention, in spite of the fog of narcotics dulling his brain. "Come in," he mumbled.

A trio of middle-aged officers walked in, uniforms perfect in every way. *A lot different from what I saw in Iraq*, he thought.

He struggled to sit up, but one of them put his hand on Samuel's shoulder. "Stay put, soldier. You don't need to move. We just have some questions for you."

His gaze ran over the three men, a puzzled frown creasing his brow. Had he done something wrong? He nodded silently, encouraging them to continue.

"How are you getting along?" one asked.

"All right, Sir." His speech slurred and Samuel hoped he didn't sound drunk.

"Is there anything you need? Anything we can do for you?" asked another.

"Thank you, Sir, but I'm doing okay."

The senior officer didn't look convinced. "Good. Well, then, we need you to tell us what you remember about the bomb."

Samuel shook his head. "I don't, Sir. Remember that is. It . . . uh . . . happened so fast, I didn't have time to think."

He shrugged. "I heard the explosion, flew back against the building, and the next thing I knew, they were carting us all off."

"Don't you remember pulling the others from the vehicle? You're a hero, Son," the senior officer said.

"No, Sir. I just did my job. I was buying fresh food for the soldiers. That's all I know." He turned his head away from them and stared out the window. "I need to rest, Sir. If you don't mind."

"All right, Samuel. We'll talk again later."

They quietly left the room, and Samuel turned back in time to see the door slowly close behind them. What the hell did they want? he wondered. He'd received a letter from the Department of the Army. Something about a medal of valor. He didn't want one. He wanted his life back. He tried to move his fingers and couldn't. They had managed to save them, the doctors said. But what good were they if he couldn't use his hand. And it was his right hand, too. The one he used for everything.

Now his military career was over, and he wasn't sure how he could be a cook, much less a chef, with only one good hand.

The sadness and hopelessness hit him without warning, as it had more and more often over the last two weeks. Despair threatened to clog his airways, and he fought to suck air into his lungs. His ribs weren't so sore now as they had been. The four ribs that were shattered in the bomb blast were healing, he could tell. But his heart, that was another thing. He couldn't work construction with his dad, couldn't even chop vegetables with one hand out of commission. What the hell did he think he was going to do for a living?

He reached over and pushed the button on his automatic pain medicine pump, allowing more morphine to run into his IV tube. Within minutes, he felt drowsiness take over as he drifted into a drug induced sleep.

John talked to his older son, Ramon, in the hall outside Samuel's room. "What are we going to do, Ramon? He seems to be slipping away from us."

Ramon frowned at his father, rubbing an ache behind his eyes. "What do the doctors say?"

John snorted. "They think he needs a psychiatrist and a special program of treatment. They think he's got some psychological problem."

"He probably does have some adjustments to make with all of this. The nurses told me he wakes up screaming that he can't get everyone out. That men are dying." He shook his head. "It's almost as though he doesn't believe everyone survived. Colonel Morrison said he wouldn't even tell them about saving the others. Claimed he didn't remember any of it."

"So what are we going to do?"

"I finish my final internship in transpersonal psychology in a couple of weeks. I could work with him, do some counseling."

"I thought you were coming home to work. You can't be coming down here all the time."

"I am," Ramon said. "I've been hired to work with the substance abuse program." He hesitated looking at Samuel's door, as though able to see through it to his brother beyond. "What if we take him home?"

"His doctors say they won't release him yet. He needs physical therapy and more surgery on his hand first."

Ramon shrugged. "I don't know how good it is for him to be here. They told me he freaked out in physical therapy yesterday. It seems to bother him to see the other wounded soldiers. It makes him really anxious, to a point they have to stop and bring him back to his room."

"I know, they mentioned it to me, too. They want us to talk him into going into the psychiatric ward to become part of some new program they are testing. They say it's the only way to help him, and there are only two places left in the first group."

"What he needs is to come home to his people. They don't know him like we do," Ramon snapped. Samuel was five years younger than he, and he was determined to protect him now, like he couldn't when his brother was in Iraq.

"They say the treatment is both medical and psychological. That it can help him heal. They didn't tell me anymore. Just he has to do it."

"He doesn't need that. He needs a traditional healing ceremony by a haatali and then counseling that I can give him. We can take turns bringing him down here for physical therapy if we have to. Maybe I can find someone on the rez to do it."

"I don't know, Ramon. What about all his painkillers and things? How will we get those?"

"We need to help him so he can stop taking so much or he is going to end up addicted. We have to get back our Sam. Now he is in a constant daze with or without the drugs. It's like no one is home, he isn't at peace. We need to get him to a place where he can balance body, mind, and spirit again. That is on the reservation, his home."

John paced back and forth twice, then stopped and looked earnestly at Ramon. "All right. I believe you know what you are doing. I will support this. How do we get him out of here?"

"We get him to agree to sign himself out AMA."

"What's that?" John asked.

"Against medical advice. They won't like it, but they don't have to. He can sign himself out if he wants to. We'll bring him back for the surgeries and do the rest of his recovery at home."

"Let's get it done then. I want to get him home as soon as we can." John turned and led Ramon into Samuel's room, determined to convince him to come home. His family and his people would take care of him there.

It didn't work. Samuel was afraid to leave. As much as he wanted to get away from the evidence of war he saw in the other soldiers, he didn't think he could go home yet, either. Besides, not accepting the new treatment would be like disobeying an order. So he refused the help John and Ramon offered and stayed in the hospital to continue to mend as well as he could.

By the third week, Samuel was more ready to leave. His hand was recovering from additional surgery and physical therapy, but the psychological symptoms persisted. Someone dropping a medical chart on the floor would have him diving for cover, and it was a rare night that he didn't awaken screaming in terror. The nurses had told him he cried out, "Save them! Don't run. I can't get them out alone!" Ramon had convinced him, though, that to heal he needed to be among the Navajo, home on his land and with his people.

As John pulled away from the hospital, Samuel glanced over his shoulder almost wishing he could stay forever. He felt safe there, and he had ready access to painkillers. Going home would give him one thing he didn't have here, though — solitude. He could think and just be for awhile. After all, there wasn't much else he could do anyway until his hand healed, if it healed.

Months passed and Ramon worked with Samuel a couple of times a week. The tribal elders had joined Ramon and the Shaman in a sweat lodge ceremony with Samuel and during traditional healing rituals. Everyone wanted the old happy Samuel back. They expected Ramon to help his brother heal quickly.

Samuel spent his days walking on the plateaus, emptying his mind and heart, trying to find peace. It wasn't working. The nightmares continued, and Samuel became agitated during any drives they had to take to the VA hospital or anywhere else off the reservation. Once when they passed a burned out car on the highway, Samuel had become terribly distraught and demanded they return to the reservation, skipping his medical appointment.

Ramon sat across from Samuel in their family home. The room was small, so his parents had taken a drive to town to leave them alone.

"How are you, Samuel?"

He shrugged and held up his still mostly useless hand. "How do you think?" He sounded bitter, something Ramon had never known him to be.

"I thought you had regained some use of your fingers — that it was getting better each week."

"It's better, but not good enough to use for anything." His voice was dejected, and he refused to look Ramon in the eye.

Ramon felt his own spirits falter. He'd been so sure he could help Samuel. His parents and the village elders were counting on him to help his brother, to bring him back from the brink of disaster. His mind raced, reviewing the work they had done, questioning what else he could say or do to ease his brother's misery.

"Samuel, we are all here to help you. To get you through this."

Samuel shook his head, his chin dropping onto his chest as he refused to meet Ramon's gaze.

"There has to be something I can do. I have studied and trained for this kind of help. What is it you need? How can I help you heal?"

"You cannot. I don't believe I am meant to heal in the way you mean. I am trapped in my own personal hell. All because I tried to do what was right."

"You didn't try. You did. You got those men out, won a medal of valor. They would have died without you."

"Then why was I punished by taking away my physical abilities?"

"You know we don't believe in a punishing Spirit. Why do you say such a thing, Samuel?"

"Because it is true. I didn't believe in that kind of god until now. Now I know the truth."

Feeling a deep sense of despair, Ramon lifted his hands and then dropped them into his lap. "How can I help you, Brother? I am at a loss here."

Samuel slowly got to his feet. "I think only time and the Great Creator can help, no one else can. And I don't think he wants to heal me."

Ramon watched his beloved younger brother walk from the cabin, his head hanging, cradling his hand in front of his chest. Ramon slammed his fist against the table that had been between the two brothers and cursed the fate that had brought this on Samuel. Then he cursed himself for being helpless to fix everything for him.

Ethical Points to Consider:

In this case, we find an example of ethical codes applying to research. Research ethics exist to protect the rights of participants. Ethics codes require participation without coercion (ACA, 2005; APA, 2002; & NASW, 2008). Participants are provided with informed consent. Among other things, this includes understanding the risks and benefits of participating in the study (ACA, 2005; APA, 2002; & NASW, 2008). Moreover, participants must be presented with any alternative treatments. An understanding of what the study consists of, length of time involved, and what participants will be doing, is necessary. In rare instances where deception is involved, participants must be debriefed following the research (ACA, 2005; APA, 2002; & NASW, 2008). For research involving deception, review boards carefully weigh whether the deception outweighs the benefits, and that the risks to participants are minimal. These guidelines exist to ensure participation is voluntary. In many settings, human research boards, review proposed studies for ethical compliance and approve the protocols prior to the research commencing.

Professional practices and ethical codes also caution against dual relationships, such as seeing one's relatives, friends, spouses, and children as a client in therapy (ACA, 2005; APA, 2002; NAADAC, 2008; & NASW, 2008). These cautions exist because of the difficulty of maintaining therapist objectivity while having a secondary relationship with the client.

Discussion Questions:

1. What cognitions, emotions and behaviors are apparent in Samuel? Given these, would you recommend treatment? Formulate a treatment plan using a theoretical orientation that you believe would be effective in this case.

2. What disorder(s) does Samuel exhibit when admitted to the hospital? What disorder(s) does Samuel exhibit at the end of the case?

3. Ramon understands Sam and his culture, which motivates him to take Samuel home. What are the positives and negatives of his actions and pressures? Assume Ramon is not his brother, but a licensed mental health professional with 20 years experience. Does your viewpoint change? Explain.

4. How would you balance Ramon's desire to help Samuel, the importance of community, cultural factors, and ethical codes?

5. What should be done about the new treatment if it truly is the best current option available according to the hospital? Assume that the new treatment is now nine months old and showing excellent results across multiple measures and multiple participant

pools. Does your viewpoint change? Explain and discuss whether the wait and quality of life issues were worth it.

6. Assume Samuel wanted to return to fighting and the military allowed it. How would your opinions on war impact your exploring this option with Samuel or signing a fitness for duty form?

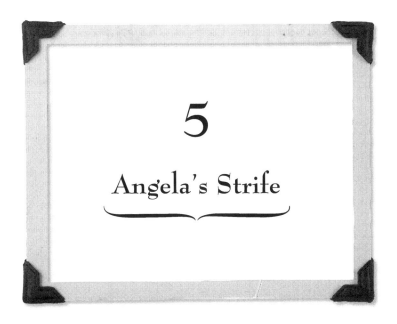

5

Angela's Strife

For Your Consideration

As you read the following case, consider the many layers of Angela's life and how these varied layers impact her currently. How do family, personal life, and her work culture contribute or help?

Angela's Story

When her name was called, Angela walked to the front of the room and shook hands with John Wilson, her supervisor. He handed her a small gold pin with the number 15 in the center. The tiny ruby sparkled at the center, making her think of a star — one that was burning out. The smile she plastered on for photographs quickly faded as sadness enveloped her. She'd had such high expectations for herself, and they seemed to be slipping away.

This job was everything she ever wanted when she graduated from Florida State University. She'd pursued a job on the factory line and worked her way up to Materials Manager. Her gaze slid around the crowded room, over people who lost a day's pay if she failed in her job. No parts, no work. The entire process fell on her shoulders. Angela sighed. Any delays caused by her cost not only the company money, but these workers as well. And heaven knew they couldn't afford to miss work anymore than she could.

She walked the perimeter of the room, an untouched piece of chocolate cake in her trembling hand. Angela stopped in front of a man with thinning hair and a growing belly. "Congratulations, Ted. Twenty-five years here is impressive."

"Thanks, so is fifteen. You'll get your twenty-five year pin one day, too." As he stuffed a large bite of cake into his mouth she wandered away, heavy at heart. Twenty-five years here? Could she last another ten, five or even one?

She walked up to another recipient to congratulate her, the smile on her face feeling false and a bit thin. "Jenny, congratulations. You've done really well here in five years. Made a lot of moves up the ladder."

The blonde smiled back, appearing genuinely thrilled with herself and her work. "Thanks, Angela. Same to you. What —"

Unable to take another minute, Angela broke in. "Excuse me Jenny. I have to get back to work. Enjoy your cake," she said nodding at the woman's serving.

Dropping her cake into the trash, she swung past the punch bowl and took a cup. She gulped it down, hoping the sugary sweetness would give her a boost. With a final glance around the room, she headed out the double doors and back to work. She saw her supervisor's frown as he watched her leave and wondered what his problem was.

She had tried to put on a good face for the party. Tears welled up in her eyes, but before they could fall, she turned and walked away from the celebration.

John followed her into the hall, catching her by the elbow and gently turning her around. "What's wrong, Angela? Aren't you proud of yourself? You should be."

Angela pushed at the black braid created to control her thick, wiry hair. "Sure, John," she said quietly, her gaze on her coffee-colored hands.

"What's wrong? You haven't been yourself lately. Not for a long time really."

She opened her mouth to speak, but closed it again, unable to force a sound through her closed throat. Angela just shook her head and left. She heard him call her name, but didn't turn back. This was something she had to deal with alone. There was no one else to turn to. Her parents had enough on their minds. She wasn't about to call on them for support.

"Sarah, I don't know what to do about Angela," John told the employee assistance counselor. "She's changed over the last few years. When we moved her up to materials manager, she took to it like a natural."

"So, what's changed?" the counselor asked.

"I don't know. I can't put my finger on it. I'm beginning to wonder if she's depressed. She used to go way above and beyond, determined to keep the parts in and make sure we didn't have to shut down the line and send people home." He shrugged. "She doesn't seem to care anymore."

"Do you know if anything's gone wrong at home for her?"

"She's pretty private. She hasn't shared much of a personal nature with me. I do know she lived with one of our other managers for a long time, and then he transferred out and they split up."

"I would suggest you recommend she come see me. I can't help her if she won't come in."

John nodded. "I'll talk to her today." As he got to his feet, he hesitated. "I really like Angela, and when she's on task she does a great job, but if we can't get the fire back into her, I'm going to have to consider letting her go. The discounts we have to give for late deliveries are mounting up, and the people upstairs are pressuring me to get things moving again."

"I understand. Send her in and let's see what we can do to help her."

That afternoon, Angela sat across from John. A huge oak desk filled with nicks and scratches from decades of use separated them. He leaned back in his swivel chair, fingers steepled, as he spoke to her.

"You want me to go to a counselor?" she asked quietly. "I don't need help."

"I'm worried about you, Angela." He leaned forward and rested his arms on the desktop. "On a business and a personal level. We've worked together a long time now."

"I'm fine. I just feel a little sad sometimes." Her voice was barely above a whisper and her gaze failed to meet his direct one. Actually she had been feeling down an awful lot lately, she thought.

"I don't think you're fine." He handed her a brochure about the company services. The counselor's name and number were on it. "Call and make an appointment —"

"But —"

"No but's, Angela." John got to his feet signalling the discussion was at an end. "I'm worried about you. We've gotten to be friends." He continued with a regretful tone in his voice. "But your job depends on you getting your act together. Lately we are losing too much money for late deliveries. Call Sarah Sanos; she's expecting to hear from you."

Her hands shook from the frustration and fear of losing her job; Angela accepted the brochure as she pushed up from the overstuffed chair and got to her feet. With a nod, she turned and walked out of the office.

"Damn it all. There's nothing wrong with me a good vacation can't fix," she muttered. Still, when she thought about the last couple of years, she realized she'd been slipping into some kind of a blue place. It seemed to be happening more often, and she couldn't pinpoint a reason for it. She used to love coming to work, interacting with the employees, attending meetings, and brainstorming solutions to problems. Now she recognized with a sinking feeling, she was part of the problem. She just didn't have her old spirit and energy. But it wasn't gone, just toned down. She certainly wasn't crazy and wasn't that who counselors were for? She shook her head to clear the thoughts.

Blast. Guess I'm going to a shrink anyway, crazy or not.

Angela twisted her hands together, linking and unlinking her fingers, while she waited to be called into the counselor's office. She didn't really need a professional. Lots of people had sad times in their lives. She was no different. It would pass. She'd had faith in God when she was a child in a small, all African-American Baptist church in her hometown of Birmingham. She'd gotten away from attending services regularly. Maybe that was all she needed, something new and different, she thought.

"Angela."

She jumped as the counselor's voice jerked her out of her reverie. "That's me." She hurried to her feet and followed the woman down a long hall to her office. It was small, but comfortable looking. Very cozy and friendly, Angela supposed most would consider it.

"Sit wherever you like. Let's chat a bit."

Angela picked a deep burgundy chair, sinking into the comforting arms of it. She waited silently, not knowing what to say.

"My name is Sarah Sanos. It's great to meet you. I saw you receiving your fifteen-year pin at the ceremony. Congratulations."

Angela shrugged. "It's nice, I guess. But thanks." She didn't return the "good to meet you" because she wasn't sure about that yet. At least the therapist was an African-American too.

"I've worked for this company for six years as an Employee Assistance Counselor. John came by and suggested you and I meet. Is that okay with you, Angela?"

"Looks like it has to be, doesn't it?"

"Not really. I can't help if you don't want me to."

Angela thought of the blue days, the loneliness lately. Maybe this woman could help. "Let's see what happens," she said.

"Fair enough. Tell me how you are, and what I can do to help you."

They went through the conversation with John and his concerns for Angela.

"I don't think anything's really wrong," she said. "Isn't it normal to feel a bit down sometimes?"

"It is, yes. We all have those days, but if you have too many it begins to impact your daily living."

Angela dropped her chin onto her chest as her voice lowered. "You mean like my job performance."

Sarah nodded. "Yes, like that and your personal life, too. Your relationships with friends and loved ones. How are those relationships working for you?"

Angela shrugged. When she thought about it, she had no personal relationships, not really. Her work was her life. No boyfriend, no special girl friends to run around with. She sighed; she even felt distanced from her parents in spite of calling them every week. Oftentimes the calls were stilted because of the tension that occasionally rose between her parents following their second try at marriage.

"Hate to say it, but I really don't have any. I go to work I go home. That's it."

"Don't you want to have relationships outside of work?"

"I used to," Angela said.

"All right. Let's take a look at that. Can we start with your family?"

Angela shrugged. "I'm an only child, so there really wasn't ever much of anyone around."

"What about your parents?" Sarah asked, jotting an occasional note.

"Mom was busy as a surgical nurse. When I got older, I watched her work from the gallery a few times. It was cool, but I didn't want a job around that much blood." She let her voice trail off.

"And your father," Sarah encouraged.

"Dad worked at the bank. When I was a kid he approved business loans, so wherever we went in town, he knew someone. Over the years, he moved into management and then just knew the heavy hitters who we never saw. I missed all the free sodas, ice creams and things his loan customers gave me when I went around town with him."

"Was that all you missed? The treats?"

Angela shook her head with a sigh. "No. I missed spending time with him. I had great fun with Dad and the customers."

"How was it when you were with both your parents?"

"Great, as long as it was only one of them at a time. When they were together, they fought a lot. In fact, they married, divorced, and then remarried. They live in the retirement community downtown now."

"How has your relationship history been? Boyfriends, girlfriends?"

"I dated Jerry from high school till I finished college. We lived together and it was good. I wouldn't really say it was wonderful. It was more just comfortable. We ended things after college to follow our careers." She tipped her head to the side thinking back. "The only other one was Mark. He worked for the copier division — that was before you started here. Anyway, we dated and lived together for about five years. He was switched to the new plant when it was finished. The fifty-mile commute got old, especially when he started staying there during the week and only coming home on weekends. I guess it just didn't work out. He wanted other things — a wife, kids. I wanted a career. I got so busy at work and trying to move up in the company, I let my personal life go." She quirked an eyebrow. "I guess I just don't care anymore. Relationships take too much work, and I have other things to do. I don't want to get married, so why pursue a relationship that won't go anywhere?"

The two women talked a bit longer, then Sarah set her tablet and pen aside. "I think we need to talk about some of these issues you've shared with me. Things seem to be out of balance in your world, and you should sort through them so you can go forward again."

The sadness felt heavy to Angela when she thought about what was missing in her life and the road it had taken. But she could keep going on. She wasn't crazy, and she certainly didn't need drugs. On the other hand, she wasn't as excited to get up and go to work as she used to be. Things were just a bit askew lately in her part of the world. Perhaps Sarah could help after all.

Four weeks later, Angela slumped in the easy chair in Sarah's office.

"We're not getting anywhere," Angela said in frustration. "I can't get a decent night's sleep. I'm not really sad, but I'm always down. I'm ready to give up."

"Perhaps we need to consider clinical depression," Sarah suggested.

"No! I'm not depressed. I'm just a little sad."

"Tell me again how long you have felt like this?"

"It seems like forever, but maybe three years. All I need is a vacation, but work gets in the way."

"How's work going these days?"

Angela shrugged. "If I go away, the production line might shut down and people go home without pay. So I work. I've tried to focus so the production output stays on schedule, but it doesn't seem to help. It just isn't as exciting as it used to be."

"What can we do to turn this around?"

"I don't know." Angela jumped to her feet and paced in front of Sarah's chair. "Maybe I should quit and go sell shoes someplace."

"I don't think you have to take it that far," Sarah said with a gentle smile on her lips. "But we do need to get you back to enjoying your work if you are going to stay there."

"I don't think they want me anymore. I don't know whether I want to be there, even." Angela shook her head. "I can't do this today. I have work to get to," she said tearfully. "I'm just a bit down."

"Angela," Sarah called out to her as Angela hurried from the office. She had a good job, nice apartment. Everything was going according to plan. Maybe this is all there is to life. This is it. People only laugh and find it exciting in the movies. Angela hurried into her car and drove toward the plant. She had a job to do.

"Sarah, how's it going with Angela?" John asked.

With the ethics training she'd had at the university, Sarah was still not comfortable with discussing an employee's status. But she was paid by the company, so she did have a certain loyalty to them.

She shook her head. "She's in a real slump. I can't seem to help her get out of it. I think it is going to take some time for her to work through her issues, if she can."

He got to his feet. "I can't wait that long. The big bosses are pressuring me to let her go or to demote her to the production line."

"I hate to see you do that, John. It won't help her state of mind."

"I can't help it. If you can't give me some hope that she's going to snap out of this soon, it will be taken out of my hands."

Sarah thought of Angela, of her need for this job, and what losing it would do to her. The company hired Sarah to handle employee issues for them, though. She huffed out a breath, then looked John right in the eye.

"In my professional opinion, it will take several months to help Angela work through this period in her life. As with all clients, there is never a guarantee of success."

"Thanks, Sarah. I guess I know what I have to do then."

He turned and left her office, leaving Sarah with a heavy feeling around her heart.

Ethical Points to Consider:

This case points out the need for mental health professionals to carefully clarify for whom the therapist is working, to avoid conflicts of interest (ACA, 2005; APA, 2002; NAADAC, 2008; & NASW, 2008). When working with referrals from probation officers and the courts, for example, there generally is a mandate to report back to the referral source. This could include number of sessions attended by the client and material discussed by the client. Often, the report is limited to the number of sessions and whether progress is being made. The client needs to understand prior to therapy what will be reported, and to whom. In this case study, the employer views himself as also employing the therapist and therefore having a right to information from the client's session. Employee Assistance Program counselors must carefully clarify what, if any, information is to be reported back to the company. The key in these situations is to clearly articulate and inform the client regarding all information that will be reported, to whom, and how frequently.

Discussion Questions:

1. Currently, what cognitions, emotions, and behaviors are having the most influence on Angela? Given these, what theoretical orientation will guide your work with her? How do you conceptualize the case?
2. What impact does diversity have?

3. Would you diagnose Angela; and if so, with what? What are your thoughts regarding referring Angela for medication evaluation?

4. Who is the client in this case? What ethical demands does the therapist need to balance? How would you sort out and address the competing demands?

5. What would be your initial treatment plan?

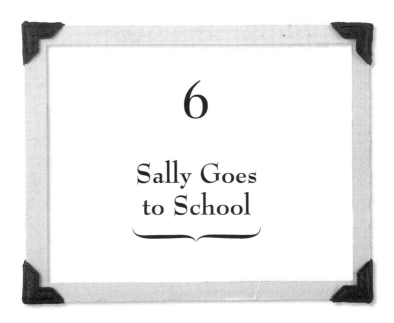

6

Sally Goes to School

For Your Consideration

As you read the following case, consider what Sally's parents are experiencing. How do parents' dreams and hopes for their child impact their observations and conclusions? What options are available? How would the options for Sally vary depending on culture, location, and economics?

Sally's Story

Lisa watched in fear as her daughter, Sally, rocked on the preschool floor. Her tiny body curled tightly into a fetal position, her small fists clenched and held against her body. Her muscles were tensed, looking as though they could snap, even though she rocked back and forth.

"What's happening?" Lisa asked. The teacher led her to the girl and together they bent down to try and break into the child's trancelike state.

"She does this several times a week. We've tried to explain, but you and your husband don't want to hear it. Sally needs help."

Lisa reached a hand out to run her fingers up and down Sally's arms, then tried unsuccessfully to pull her into an embrace. "What kind of help?" she whispered.

"I'm not sure. I'd start with the pediatrician and follow her recommendations."

Lisa tried again to lift her daughter, but the stiffness of her body made it difficult. Sally seemed to become even more upset by the attempts, and began to bang her head against the tile floor. When Lisa reached toward her again, the teacher stopped her. "All we can do is slide a pillow under her head and wait for it to pass. Unless you want to call an ambulance?"

She thought of her child being hauled into an ambulance, of the fear that could result, and shook her head. "As long as you think she's breathing okay and everything, let's wait a minute. Does it usually take long to pass?"

"Not usually. A few minutes that seem like hours." She offered a reassuring smile to Lisa, but Lisa could only focus on her baby's horrible situation. What can I do to help her? she wondered. Fear gnawed at her belly and left her weak-kneed. How can I bring my child back from such a precipice? she wondered.

Psychologist Carl Rain glanced from the papers on his desk to the couple across from him who were referred by their pediatrician. Lisa and Jack Watterton sat close together, their hands clasped, knuckles white. Beside them, in a large chair that seemed to dwarf her body, sat their daughter, Sally. She was turning a small stuffed toy over and over in her hands, determinedly ignoring the rest of them.

"According to this, Sally's preschool has refused to keep her. They seem to think she has a problem. Can you tell me what's been happening?"

Jack stayed quiet, so Lisa spoke up. "I don't know exactly. At the school the other day, I stopped to pick her up and she was having a . . . a meltdown I guess you could call it."

"How do you mean that, Mrs. Watterton? What was she doing exactly?"

Carl listened carefully and jotted notes as the girl's mother described the scene at the school.

"Are you aware of any particular pattern to these 'meltdowns'?"

"I'm not sure." She shrugged and pulled her hand from Jack's to raise both, and then drop them helplessly into her lap. She picked up a tissue there and twisted it mercilessly in her fingers. "The teachers seem to think it happens most when the routine changes. Apparently, she doesn't like that. They said she doesn't like to share, either." The woman looked at Carl imploring for understanding.

"She's not like this at home. Something is wrong at that place. Maybe I should just keep her home and home school her."

Jack snorted. "That's not going to do anything and you know it. Something's wrong with her."

Carl noted the father didn't seem overly concerned. "Is she your only child, Mr. Watterton?"

"Yeah, she is." His gaze drifted to his daughter and he seemed to go back in time. "We were so excited when she was born. Not only was she our first, she was the first grandchild." He said then, lightening his own mood a bit, "She must have had a thousand pictures taken of her when she was born, before she came home. And after . . . well, who could count."

"You sound very proud of her," Carl commented.

"We were . . . are" Jack shook his head, lost for a moment in thought.

"Have you had any problems with babysitters, like you do the school?"

"Yes, we have. We can't really find anyone willing to stay with her anymore. One of us is with her all the time now," Lisa said. "I quit my job and work at home as a seamstress to bring in extra money. Jack works in construction and is gone long hours during good weather."

"How is Sally in her development? She seems a bit small for her age. Is she able to do things you think other three- and four-year-olds do?"

"Mostly," Jack answered. "She does need help getting dressed. Tying her shoes and zipping things up. But, she's really smart," he said proudly.

"Oh? In what ways?"

"She knows the theme songs to most of the kid's television shows by heart. She can sing 'em well, too." Jack shifted in his seat to look at Sally. "Sally, why don't you sing the doctor a pretty song? . . . Sally?"

The girl kept turning her toy over, closely inspecting it and showing no indication she had heard a word from her father. He sighed and leaned back. "Well, when she's on her own at home, she walks around singing to herself all the time."

Lisa spoke up. "She walks around whispering to herself, too. Is that normal, Dr. Rain?"

Carl ignored her for the moment. "What about her sleep patterns?"

The bags under Lisa's eyes pretty much told that story, but he needed to hear it from them. "She doesn't stay down. She's up and down all night, and so am I. She tosses and turns all night. She insists on wearing one pair of warm pajamas even in the summer, so she gets hot and throws the sheets off. I worry she's going to get sick that way."

"Is she particular about other things, too?"

"I wouldn't say particular, just independent. That's because she's an only child," Jack said.

"In what ways does she show her independence?"

"Well, she hates shoes, but that's because they hurt her feet."

"Does she makes friends at school?"

Lisa shook her head. "No. She's really independent like Jack said. She plays alone, entertaining herself most of the time."

"She avoids interactions with strangers, but that's just because she understands stranger danger. We worked hard to teach her that so no one can hurt her," Jack added.

Carl leaned back and pulled some forms from his lower desk drawer. "I'd like to have you sign a release so I can visit the school, perhaps get them to allow her to come for a day or two so I can observe. I'd also like to talk to anyone else in the family that spends time with her. Who would that be?"

"Probably my sister more than anyone. Melanie Beale. Our parents haven't known how to deal with Sally, so they don't see her as much as they used to."

"If you'd sign these releases, we'll move to the next step."

"And what is the next step?" Jack asked.

"I'd like to have Sally do a psychoeducational assessment and neuro-logical evaluation."

"But why?" Lisa burst out. "She's only a little behind the others. We can work this out, I'm sure."

"It's routine, Mrs. Watterton. We'll rule out any physiological problems and have a better idea exactly where Sally is in her development. With your permission?" He glanced from mother to father and back, watched as they looked at each other and then their daughter.

Finally Jack said, "All right. What do we do?"

"Ms. Beale, thanks for coming. Have a seat."

Carl sat next to the young woman and crossed his legs. "What can you tell me about your niece, Sally?"

"She's beautiful, but I'm guessing that's not what you're after."

"Yes, she is, and no, it's not. What do you know about her behavior lately?"

"She doesn't seem to like to interact with anyone. No playmates, especially no strangers." Tears well in her eyes, suddenly gone sad. "She won't even interact with my parents. They were so excited about having a grandchild. They took tons of pictures, spent hours picking out things for her. Now she won't even acknowledge them if they are in the same room."

"Have you seen her episodes?"

A silent nod.

"When have you seen this?"

"Hmmm . . . when we use a different baby sitter . . . when she has to do something the way we want, instead of the way she wants."

Carl glanced up from his notes. "Anyone in particular she does well or poorly with?"

"She has trouble with anyone new, but she seems especially upset around people with hats. I suppose she can't see their faces. Come to think of it, she is as nervous around everyone."

"What have you thought about how she acts?"

"Well, at first I thought we had spoiled her. You know, all the attention and everything. But now I'm not sure. It seems to go way beyond that or having a temper. I've seen kids throw a temper fit, and what she does looks really different from that."

"Do you know anything about how she is at the preschool?"

"Only that she hasn't made friendships there. She plays alone, doesn't share her toys." Melanie shrugged. "That sort of thing."

"Anything else you can tell me?"

"Only that we're all really worried. She seems to be withdrawing more each year instead of coming out of her shell. We don't know what to do to help her. Can you help her?"

"I think so, Melanie." They both rose. "Thanks for coming. You've been a great help."

Melanie nodded and walked from the room, digging a tissue from her purse. Carl knew the impact a child like Sally could have on the whole family. She wouldn't be the only one in the family who needed some counseling help.

A couple of weeks later, Jack and Lisa walked into Carl's office and had a seat. This time they had left Sally at the preschool after Carl had intervened and explained he needed to observe her there.

"I just came from the school. I saw most of the behaviors you, the teachers, and Melanie mentioned. Let's go over the test results, then we'll talk more about that."

"All right," Jack said.

"Sally has lower verbal scores with a wide scatter of scores in the subtests. She has an overall IQ of 65."

"What about the medical tests?" Lisa asked, an anxious note in her voice.

"The neurological tests were all normal. She's in the 45th percentile for height and weight." Carl flipped through the file briefly. "There doesn't appear to be any history of mental illness in the family. Right?"

"That's right. But I want actual scores and test questions," Jack answered.

"Well, let's work through this a piece at a time then. We'll get to the bottom of it." Dr. Rain gave them a reassuring smile and turned once more to the file.

"As long as I get the questions and scores."

Ethical Points to Consider:

In this case, the parents are demanding not only test results but also access to test questions and individual question scores. The APA (2002) code of ethics requires psychologists to conduct adequate assessment and evaluation upon which they base diagnosis and reports. Here information was gathered from the parents, aunt and through observation of the child in her school setting. The psychologist was careful to gather informed consent from the parents for everything he was doing. The child's parents demanded her answers, scores, and a copy of the assessment questions. APA (2002) ethics allow for releasing the child's answers to the questions and all scores (raw and scaled). However, the codes (APA) prohibit release of test materials, including actual test questions. Psychologists have a duty to protect test materials from release, in order to prevent assessment questions from becoming publicly available and invalidating the tests. For example, if the questions on IQ tests were known to the child's parents they could coach her in the correct answers. If IQ questions were available to the public, some individuals seeking to represent themselves with higher or lower scores would answer in ways to seek personal gain, such as receiving social security disability or gaining admittance into a private school/society based on IQ.

Discussion Questions:

1. What behaviors, cognitions, and emotions of Sally's are unusual? Given these, what, if any, diagnosis(es) do you find?

2. What part of her not "interacting" is typical for a child and centers on the parents' expectations?

3. What problems is Sally experiencing that could be normal developmental delays in particular, given her assessment results?

4. How would you conceptualize the case and from what theoretical orientation? Describe the potential benefits/risks of family therapy.

5. How does the school impact this case?

6. What adjuncts to therapy would you recommend?

7. How would you handle convincing the school to take Sally back so that an observation of her school behavior can be completed?

8. What steps are necessary and appropriate to facilitate gathering information about Sally?

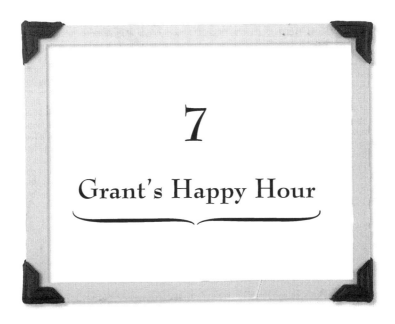

7

Grant's Happy Hour

For Your Consideration

As you read the following case, be aware of your biases and reactions to Grant's diversity. How do your reactions and assumptions about Grant's friend impact your empathy and assessment of the situation?

Grant's Story

"Grant Alexander," Bill called out. He watched a sullen-looking man rise and come toward him. The mid-thirties man wore Dockers, loafers, and a resentment-filled frown. This one's going to take a while, Bill thought. He put a smile on his own face. "Right this way, Mr. Alexander."

Grant followed him into a large office and dropped into an over-stuffed recliner.

Bill sat opposite and opened the file in his hands. "Why don't you tell me why the courts saw fit to send you to me?"

He shrugged. "DUI. It was this or jail."

He didn't sound too sure which would be worse.

"Before we get to that, why not tell me a bit about your family."

"Not much to tell." Grant tipped his head to the side as though looking back in time. "Dad was a miner."

"Here in Alaska?"

"No, lower forty-eight — Virginia, actually. Mom taught school in the small mining town we lived in."

"Sibs?"

"Two. A brother who was the football hero of our town, Mr. Macho, and a sister who was such a prissy daddy's girl it was pathetic."

Bill watched Grant cross his legs and swing one foot, the speed increasing as he talked about the family.

"Was your brother older or younger?"

"Older. They were always trying to compare me to him. Thought I should go out for football, too." He scoffed at that.

"What about schooling?"

"I have a bachelor's in mining engineering."

"Did you drink at college?"

"What frat brat doesn't? We spent our weekends partying." He shrugged. "It helped me relax and have fun. When I'd had a couple, I could ask people to dance and stuff. If I didn't have any booze, I just kept to myself while everyone else had fun."

"Did you drink every day?"

Grant shook his head. "No, I held it to weekends so I could get through my classes during the week. Then I drank like crazy, drinking from Thursday night till Sunday and then going to class Monday with the mother of all hangovers."

"Have you ever tried to stop?"

"Didn't see any reason to."

Bill wasn't sure this patient was ready for help. He sighed and then asked Grant to tell him what had happened. "Tell me about the arrest. What were you doing just before that?"

Grant stared into space for a full minute, the silence in the room growing taut enough to snap. With a shrug, he began to tell his story.

"Sam and I walked into a bar filled with smoke. Kind of a local hangout. Loud music, laughter, and the crack of billiard balls met us at the door. We had come to throw darts, so we walked to the back of the bar, calling out a greeting to the bartender as we passed him."

"Hey, Ted, bring us a couple of beers, would you?" I asked. "My voice was slurred, so I glanced at my watch wondering how long we'd been at it. We'd been drinking beer since ten that morning, and it was past eight in the evening. I couldn't remember if we'd ever eaten lunch or dinner." Grant shook his head as though still disbelieving the day went down the way it had.

"What do you remember next?"

"As we weaved through the crowd toward the game boards, one of the guys grabbed Sam and handed over the microphone to the Karaoke equipment.

"All I wanted was to dive into another beer, but I knew Sam liked to belt out the songs. When the song was done, I clapped and whistled, then led the way to the dartboard.

"I told Sam that was enough screwin' around. I wanted to throw darts."

"What did Sam want to do?"

"Sam just laughed and asked if I thought we could still hit the wall, let alone the board. Sam guessed we'd guzzled a few cases worth of beer that day."

"What did you think?" Bill asked looking up from his notepad.

"I was fine." Grant shrugged. "When I looked at the board, I really had to work at focusing on it. I told Sam I wanted to get started. I was ready to kick ass. I picked up the darts and handed the blue ones to Sam.

"Later that night we stumbled home, and Sam went straight to bed. Too much beer, I guess. At home, Sam drinks white wine. Anyway, I suppose I wasn't ready to stop. I took a new, chilled bottle and stepped out onto the porch with an extra beer in my other hand. Darkness surrounded the cabin. The cold snapped in the air, even though it was still late summer." He shivered at the memory.

"I remember it was really cold, so I reached back inside and grabbed a light weight jacket off a hook, draped it across my shoulders and dropped onto a porch swing to drink. I was thinking about my family in the lower forty-eight, knew they'd disapproved of me all the way around." Grant lifted his hands, palm up and then dropped back into his lap. "Guess I was kind of wallowing in self-pity at that point. I chugged the beer and reached beside me to pick up and twist the cap off another. I'd always had competition from my brother and sister. Never been quite good enough for Mom and Dad. Daddy's Girl and Football Hero, that's the way I thought of my brother and sister. Mr. and Ms. Perfect. Could do no wrong. And then there was me."

"And what about you do you think your father didn't like?"

"Everything. I never liked sports. Didn't see any sense to running down a field carrying a ball so a bunch of bruisers could land on top of me, just to get it back. I was intellectual and enjoyed my studies; belonged in Geeksville, I guess.

"I just kept drinking beer that night. Couldn't get enough of it to drown my thoughts. My father had never approved of me and my disinterest in sports. A retired miner, I knew they didn't come much tougher than my old man. My mother was more gentle and accepting, but she followed Dad's lead. If he disapproved, she followed along, somewhat apologetic about it in the process.

"College was a challenge for me. I made it though. I remember holding the beer bottle that night in Juneau and reading the label. It triggered a memory of the frat house. I realized I'd been a drinker then, too. But it was different. I was a weekend drinker. I can handle my booze, I'm not a drunk, I work at my job, I pay my bills, no way am I a bum. What's wrong with a few drinks after work. I don't hurt anybody, I just want to be left alone. So what, I drink a little bit every day, sometimes more than a little. I don't hurt anybody.

"The thoughts as I sat on that porch bothered me, so I just chugged the rest of my beer and staggered inside, to fall across the bed and drop into oblivion."

"So that wasn't the night you were arrested, obviously. How did that happen?" Bill asked.

"That Sunday evening, after a weekend of playing cards, drinking more beer, and telling stories, Sam and I headed for town. We'd decided it was time to go into town for a meal and more beer. We hadn't been able to carry enough in the small car to last the week we planned to stay at the cabin."

Grant felt disgust roll through him at the memory. "I climbed behind the wheel of my car, and we headed for town. I shook my head to clear it and fought to focus on the white lines that seemed to be weaving in front of my red Toyota. I kept muttering under my breath, wishing I hadn't had that last beer before driving." Grant snorted. "Like that would have made a difference. Anyway, I thought it was too late then to do anything about it and kept going.

"Sam's head drooped against the window, and a soft, rhythmic snore filled the little car. Made me smile . . ." His voice drifted away to another time and place.

"Suddenly, I noticed a police car, lights flashing behind us. I yelled at Sam to wake up; said we had big trouble. Sam looked through the rear window and asked what we were gonna do."

Grant shrugged. "Wasn't much we could do at that point but pull over. So I stopped on the side of the road. I reached for my license and registration as the officers came up, one on each side of the car." A shudder slid over him. He'd thought at the time the officers might hurt them.

"Cop asked me to get out of the car and the other one got Sam out. I climbed out and slammed the door, leaning back against it to steady myself." He huffed out a breath. "I thought I could fool them, that I could fool myself into believing I wasn't wasted. I held out the paper work, but my hands were shaking so bad I nearly dropped it. I asked him if I was speeding.

"He wanted me to take a field sobriety test. I tried to talk my way out of it, but it didn't work. He said I could take it there or downtown."

"Obviously you failed it," Bill commented, occasionally making notes again.

"Yeah, right. Next thing we knew we were on our way to the station. Sam couldn't drive, so they took Sam, too. It was all Sam could do not to slide to the ground in a puddle beside the car.

"Anyway, I tried again to talk us out of that mess. I knew a DUI would kill my auto insurance and I couldn't afford it."

"Could you afford to kill an innocent person driving drunk?"

Grant sucked in a breath. "No, no I couldn't. I don't think I could live with that."

"If you don't quit drinking, you could one day find out."

"Well, that's why I'm here, isn't it?"

Bill shook his head. "You're here because the court said you had to be. That's not how you stop drinking. Do *you* want to stop?"

Grant thought before he answered. A good sign Bill thought, instead of just saying yes to get him off his back.

"Yes. I do, I guess. I don't know. Sam said we're over if I don't change, kind of crazy 'cuz Sam drinks too, but not as much."

"All right then. This is an eight week program. You'll be checked periodically for drugs and alcohol, come into group sessions twice a week, and see me individually a few times, too. Does that all sound good to you?"

A heavy sigh slid from Grant's body. It was obvious he knew he was on an uphill climb, but had he actually hit bottom yet? Bill wasn't sure.

"Sounds good. I can do it."

The two men stood, shook hands. "I'll see you here on Tuesday, six in the evening."

"Okay. Thanks, thanks a lot."

End of Week One

Bill answered his phone when it rang. "Hello."

"Dr. Schneider, Mary here. I've got a positive test on one of your guys."

He took his glasses off and set them aside to rub the bridge of his nose. "Who is it?"

"Name's Grant Alexander."

"All right, I'll take care of it. Thanks." He gently replaced the receiver thinking about the progress he had thought Grant was making. Then he picked up the phone again, dialing a number he had scribbled on a small desk pad.

"Yeah?" Came a husky voice when the ringing stopped.

"Grant?"

"That's right. Who is this?" He sounded friendly, not aggressive at all.

"It's Dr. Schneider, Grant. I need to see you in my office. Can you come by?"

"Sure. When?"

"I had a cancellation. Can you come now?"

"Okay. Twenty minutes."

Hmmm, didn't sound like he had a care in the world, Bill thought. Maybe this was a mix-up.

A short time later he showed Grant into his office. He was clean, well-groomed, smiling. Not what you'd expect from someone who slipped off the wagon.

Bill told him about the test.

"But that isn't possible. I haven't had a drink since I left your office that first time. I don't understand."

"Have you used anything at all that could have caused a positive reading?"

"I don't think so." He frowned and chewed his lip. "Honest, doc, I haven't had a drink. In fact, I was sick last week so it was a good thing you had to cancel one of the classes. I was home in bed with a cold."

"How were you treating it?"

"Just over-the-counter mouthwash. You know a disinfectant one, I don't remember which it was. I thought it would help the sore throat."

Bill saw the light bulb turn on in Grant's brain.

"Damn. That crap has alcohol doesn't it?"

"It does. Do you have the list I gave you?"

He had the good graces to look sheepish. "I did, but I poured coffee all over it and didn't think it was important enough to replace. Sorry."

Bill got up and went to his file cabinet. He pulled a sheet of paper out and handed it to Grant. "Take this home and read it. It's all about hidden sources of alcohol. From now on you must avoid all of these things."

He wasn't sure if Grant drank it purposefully or if it was an accident. Time would tell. He liked Grant, but was confused by him. Did he really want to stop or was this a game?

"Right, doc. I can do it."

"All right. I'll see you next week."

Week Six

"Hi, doc. How's it goin'?"

"Great. How about you?"

"It isn't easy, but I'm making it."

"How's work?"

"Good, really busy. I took on two new jobs just last week."

Bill's gaze slid over Grant, assessing, taking in body language and posture. "Is that wise? You don't want stress to help break down your resolve."

Grant lifted one shoulder. "It keeps me from having time to think — time to think about things I don't want to."

"What kind of things, Grant? What is it you try to avoid?"

"Everything we say is confidential, right? It doesn't go in a report to the court or anything?"

"No, it's private. I only report your progress in the program."

"I . . . oh man, I don't know how to even approach this."

"Straight out usually works best."

"Okay then, I like men. I find myself looking at them and thinking about them the way men are supposed to think about women."

"How did that go over with your family and your football hero brother?"

Grant shook his head. "They don't know. That's partly why I came up here. To keep them from finding out and to try to get over those . . . interests."

"It sounds like this is a major issue for you. We need to work on that to help you stick with the program. That okay with you?"

Grant simply nodded his head and kept his gaze focused on the hands he clenched in his lap.

Week Seven

Finally, Friday night, Bill thought. He led his wife into the Lonestar Restaurant, their favorite steakhouse. As they were seated, he glanced into the bar. There, propping it up and belting back a beer was Grant.

"Damn . . . uh, sorry, Hon," he said, as she gazed at him with a question in her eyes.

They sat and ate, all while he kept one eye on Grant at the bar. He had several beers during the time they had their dinner. Bill wondered what he should do. He thought about offering Grant a ride home. He couldn't let him drive drunk and hurt someone. As a counselor in the program Grant attended, he also thought it essential that Grant knew he'd been seen breaking the agreement to refrain from alcohol.

Bill hated the feeling he had when this happened. The failure that tried to force itself into his mind. He knew he couldn't choose for anyone else, but he hated it every time one of the people in the program slipped through his grasp. When his wife drew his attention back to their dessert, he smiled at her and absently wondered what to do about giving Grant a ride home.

Ethical Points to Consider:

In this case, the mental health professional must consider not only confidentiality, but also potential risks to the public. Releases of client information, including who is or is not a client, are typically limited to times when a client signs a release, is a danger to self, danger to others, or abusing a child or vulnerable person (ACA, 2005; APA, 2002; NAADAC, 2008; & NASW, 2008). However, saying 'hello' to someone in public can potentially breach a client's privacy. If the mental health worker is observed by others (who know the person is a counselor) saying 'hello' to a 'stranger', the assumption is often made that the 'stranger' is the counselor's client. This usually automatic gesture can create awkward situations. Mental health workers should clearly discuss with their clients how they might ignore them in public to protect client privacy. Assume a counselor is seeing Mary for an extramarital affair. Her spouse, George, is unaware Mary is in counseling. If she bumps into her counselor at the mall and the counselor greets her, George may demand to know who the person addressing Mary is. Mary's privacy has been breached.

This case is complicated by Grant potentially drinking and driving. Duty to warn laws can be unclear in this area. Ideally, the bartender would stop serving Grant and call a cab. Confronting Grant, by the counselor in public, would not protect his confidentiality. Bennett, Bricklin, Harris, Knapp, VandeCreek, and Younggren (2006), point out that some states mandate reporting impaired drivers. In states without mandated reporting other options should be explored. The important point is to review state laws regarding impaired drivers and consider what to do prior to being in the situation.

Discussion Questions:

1. How do your assumptions about Sam impact your reading of the case? How would these assumptions impact therapy with Grant?
2. Would you approach Grant in the bar? Why or why not? How would you balance the desire to protect the public with client confidentiality?
3. What is your opinion regarding including Grant's family of origin in treatment?
4. What components of the drug/alcohol treatment program would you include?

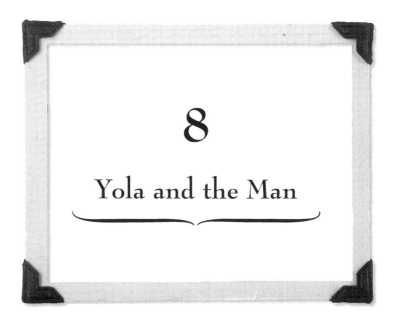

8

Yola and the Man

For Your Consideration

As you read the following case, be aware of your biases and reactions to a woman who works as a prostitute and has young children. How do your cognitive and emotional reactions impact your empathy and assessment of the situation? How do economic and cultural factors impact this case?

Yola's Story

Yola sat in the straight-backed chair across from her CPS case worker. A glance around the room showed the small blonde nearly hidden behind a stack of files on her desk. Diplomas hung on the pale green walls, and books and papers lined the wooden shelves behind her.

Yola tugged the hem of her skirt, trying to cover her bare thighs. Her scarred Caucasian skin spoke to her difficult life, and she wondered what this perfect caseworker would think of her. They all seemed snooty and judgmental to her. This one wanted to take her kids away from her. Yola just knew it.

"Are you using drugs now, Yola?" Ms. Richardson asked, looking up from the papers on her desk.

"No, I haven't used anything in a year now."

Yola could tell from the way Ms. Richardson looked at her that she didn't believe it. Well, it was mostly true, Yola thought. She had to have something to get through work. Willy pimped her on Beale Street, and she couldn't stand having a stranger's hands on her if she didn't dull the pain by smoking a little pot.

"How about alcohol?"

"Not that either." She hesitated. How honest should she be with this woman? "Well, I know I can trust you so, yes, I do have a drink now and again, like you probably do, but nothing regular. Just socially, you know?"

"What about when you were pregnant? Tell the truth now. It can help us determine how best to help Cassie and David."

Yola sighed and clasped her hands in her lap trying to stop the trembling. She needed a fix in the worst way. "I did drugs back then, but I cut back as soon as I found out I was pregnant. Both times."

"Right," Ms. Richardson muttered. "Yola, we have to consider what's in the best interest of the children. It's time to consider putting them in foster care."

Yola lunged to her feet. "No! I trusted you. You are a liar. You can't take them away from me. They're all I've got." She leaned over the desk and into Ms. Richardson's face, who leaned as far back in her chair as she could. She'd put her hand on the intercom button.

"Sit down, please."

Yola slumped onto the chair, her stomach clutching and her heart pounding. "Please, I take good care of them and when I need . . . uh . . . help, my neighbor lady feeds them a sandwich and gives them milk."

"What are you doing for work?"

"I'm a . . . a stay-at-home mom."

"We both know you can't support yourself and Cassie and David on what you get in food stamps and from public assistance. Rent is expensive. Do you have another live-in boyfriend helping you?"

"No." She looked away, afraid the caseworker would see the truth in her eyes.

"Yola, you have to be honest with me or I can't help you."

She tugged again at her skirt hem. "I haven't had many live-in boyfriends this year, only three, and this one, well, he's not a boyfriend, and he doesn't live-in. I do some work for him from time to time." She shrugged. "He pays me cash."

"Cash you don't report to your caseworker."

Yola felt mixed up. Ms. Richardson was confusing her. She didn't know whether to tell the truth or not. She stayed silent and didn't answer at all.

"What kind of work do you do for him?"

Yola didn't know why this woman was asking all these questions. She sounded like she knew everything already anyway.

"I . . . I clean houses for him . . . ."

Ms. Richardson leaned back in her chair, one eyebrow raised. "I don't believe you, I think you're back working Beale street for your old pimp."

"I swear I'm cleaning houses to keep our tiny apartment. I don't have any other skills, and I can work while the kids sleep." She rushed to say it all, to get her point across. She didn't like prostitution, but after dropping out of school it was all she knew how to do. Her adopted mom had only criticized her, but this was something she did and did well. The men never complained to Willy about her. They asked for her by name.

"What's this man's name?"

Yola felt the heat drain from her face. She didn't dare tell the authorities who he was. "I . . . ah . . . I can't say. He'd kill me," she whispered.

"And just what do you do to protect Cassie when he is there. Your last boyfriend sexually assaulted her. And you didn't believe it was physically possible, but it was. What will you do when he comes after Cassie? When he tries to take her into the business?"

"He wouldn't do that. He really loves me, not like those other jerks. No way would he do that. She's just a baby. She's six."

"I know, and I know David's only seven. He could come after the boy, too. You know they are taken into prostitution nearly as often as young girls. Do you really think the fact they are young will protect them from a man like this?"

She'd wondered the same herself, but with her drug and alcohol habit, she had to work. The only way for her to get enough to buy drugs was to hold out on Willy and pray he didn't find out. He'd beaten her so bad the last time, she'd gone to an ER to try to get help after he finished with her. Unconsciously, Yola lifted her hand and briefly touched her face before laying her hand back in her lap.

Ms. Richardson studied Yola's face closely for the first time since she'd stepped into her office. "What happened to your cheek? It looks swollen, and you've got a pile of make-up on it."

Yola lifted her hand again to gently caress the still sore bone. "I tripped going to the bus stop and fell." She shrugged. "I hit the curb pretty hard. It's better now."

Ms. Richardson shook her head. "Do you really think this is a good life for Cassie and David?" she asked gently. "Let us help you."

"They're independent and strong. I make sure they have a roof over their heads, go to school, eat . . . all that stuff."

Ms. Richardson chewed on her lip as Yola watched her. "Yola, you attempted suicide twice this year. Are you feeling ok now? Any thoughts of suicide?" The caseworker waited as the silence in the room stretched into a long pause.

Yola didn't answer. How could she?

Finally, when Yola didn't think she could stand the caseworker's silence any longer, the woman slapped Yola's file closed.

"This is what we're going to do. The counselors are going to keep seeing the children once a week. You *will* see that they get to the office on time for their appointments." She hesitated, looking at Yola questioningly.

"Yes, ma'am."

"All right then. You will stay off Beale Street and avoid all alcohol and drugs. You will show up at the local lab every 48 hours for drug screening." She stopped again.

"Yes, ma'am." Yola swallowed — hard. How did this woman think she'd survive if she did all this?

"If anything happens to further jeopardize your children, we will take them out of the home. Do you understand?"

Her heart hammered again. "Yes, ma'am."

"If this — person — hurts you or comes near your children you are to call the police immediately. Take them and go to a shelter if you need to."

Her eyes wide, Yola simply nodded, knowing if she did either of those, Willy would kill her without a second thought.

"Go on now. Get out of my office and for once, think about your children before yourself."

Yola stood on shaking legs and escaped, throwing a thank you at Ms. Richardson as she left. She'd given her another chance keep her kids. Yola had to do right by them. She had to stay clean and off the street. She ran a checklist in her head. They had some macaroni and cheese in the cabinet and some cereal, and milk in the fridge. Food money day was just three days away, so they could make it until then. But when she pictured the place she hid her drugs and scotch, all she could visualize was an empty space. And then there was Willy. He wouldn't accept her not working because of the kids. He'd put her on the street no matter what.

Yola thought briefly of taking Cassie and David and running. Where would she go? Her parents wouldn't take her in; and who knew where the kids' fathers were. No, Yola was on her own, and she knew it.

Yola made up her face in the bathroom mirror, with Cassie balanced on the edge of the tub watching. Her short blue skirt and off the shoulder blouse made her look good, she thought. Desirable. Just the way Willy wanted her to look.

Cassie pouted. "Why do you have to go out? Can't you stay home with us?"

Yola glanced in the mirror at her daughter. "I'm sorry, baby, but I have to work. We need to pay the rent and buy food."

"But you're always gone."

"I'm sorry, Cassie. I have to go. You and David watch TV and have some mac and cheese for dinner. I'll get home as soon as I can."

Cassie jumped up from the tub. "I hate you! I told Dr. Bridgett that you are always gone and I *hate* it."

Yola slowly turned to her daughter. "What else did you say to her?"

Cassie was red-faced with tears streaming down her cheeks. "I told her you're always doing drugs and you're never home! I told her we're here all by ourselves . . . alone . . ." She stuttered to a stop and hiccupped around her tears.

"Oh, baby," she reached out to Cassie, but the girl turned and ran down the short hall to her closet bedroom, slamming the door behind her.

Yola had to have a talk with that doctor. She needed to stop turning her kids against her. Yola thought about not going out, about dealing with Willy if she didn't show up for work. She might be able to withstand his fists, but could she manage without her drugs? Could she go even 24 hours without a fix? Yola knew she couldn't. She'd get through the night, and tomorrow when she took Cassie and David to see Dr. Bridgett, she'd go inside, too.

Yola stood on a corner of Beale Street, under a dim light, and watched the low slung Cadillac approach. She felt for the lump of cash in her left pocket, knowing Willy was coming to collect what she had earned so far. Maybe she could ask him to let her work fewer hours, to be home with the kids a little bit more. Maybe they could ask the customers that asked for her by name for money since they seemed to like her.

She nervously fingered the much smaller bit of cash in her right pocket, praying Willy wouldn't question the money she was about to give him. The little bit she had kept back would pay for a fix or two and a new cheap bottle of booze.

When the car door slammed, Yola jerked toward the sound and plastered a smile on her face. "Hey, Willy. How's it goin'?"

The thin, small man came around the front of the car, stepping up to Yola and pressing against her body with his own. "Great. How much you earn tonight?"

Intimidated, Yola took a step back away from the slicked down hair and cheap cologne. "It's . . . a . . . been slow tonight," she stuttered. Pulling out the roll of twenties, she handed him the bills and said, "Just a hundred and eighty."

Willy flipped through the money, counting them, and then glanced at his watch. "This all you got to show for six hours of work?"

Yola nodded silently, trying hard to keep her smile and slow her racing heart rate.

"You sure you ain't holdin' out on me, Yola? That wouldn't be smart." He stepped toward her again and caught her elbow in his free hand, squeezing it until she yelped in pain.

"No, Willy. I wouldn't do that to you. We're friends, aren't we? Besides I was gonna see if we could ask a bit more from the men who come to me all the time."

"I like the way you think. You can make even more for me that way." He stuffed the bills in his pocket and let go of her arm, distracted by her idea.

Yola gulped, steadied her voice. "I was really hoping to make the same money for you, but in fewer hours. I have to be home with my kids. Child protection is getting real edgy and talking about takin' them away from me."

Willy sighed. "Yola, Yola, now what would my other girls think if I let you do that? They'd want the same favors."

"But Willy, maybe they don't have kids. I do and I have to take care of them better or I'm gonna lose them."

The crack of his hand on her cheek, just before she tasted blood, echoed down the mostly empty road. She staggered back and caught herself before she fell. Her hand covered the heat of the slap, even as she pleaded with him.

"Willy, please don't do this. I was just asking. I can keep working if you need me."

He raised his hand as though to strike her again. She ducked and side-stepped his slow progress toward her.

A car slid around the corner and came toward them. Yola recognized the vehicle as belonging to one of her regulars. "Look, Willy. I have to go to work. They don't want damaged goods."

Willy glanced over his shoulder. "All right, get over there and take care of business. Don't be askin' for any more favors."

Tears slipped from her eyes as Yola walked to the curb, bent down to the open window and asked how she could help her customer this time. If she was lucky, she'd catch an hour or two of sleep before taking the children to their counselor.

Dr. Bridgett led both children and their mother into her office. It was fairly large, and toys were scattered over the carpeted floor. There were dolls on a table made to look like real children, and coloring books and toys designed to get children to talk about their experiences.

"Please sit down, everyone. Cassie, David, you sit wherever you want."

Yola perched on the edge of a chair, with a small table between it and the chair that Dr. Bridgett sat on.

Before Dr. Bridgett could say anything else, Yola spoke up. "You can't take my kids away, I won't allow it."

The woman was clearly agitated, and from the look of her eyes, Dr. Bridgett figured she was probably doing drugs.

"Cassie, David, why don't you go out in the front waiting area with Cheryl for a few minutes. I'd like to talk to your mother alone."

David stood and pulled Cassie to her feet. The little girl looked at Dr. Bridgett with eyes like saucers, and then looked at her mother.

"It's okay, baby. Go on out front. I'll just be a minute, and then you can come back and talk to the doctor."

The children left, quietly closing the door, as though fearing any noise would cause an explosion. Dr. Bridgett looked at Yola.

"Yola, you gave us the right to do whatever is in the best interests of the children by not caring for them yourself. You really don't have a say in the matter at this point."

"They're mine. You can't take them away." She clung to her purse, clasping it in front of her like a shield. Her knee twitched as she shook her leg up and down.

Dr. Bridgett reached toward her, intending to lay a hand on her arm, trying to calm her down. Yola jerked away from her.

"You want what's best for them, don't you?"

"I'm what's best for them. I'm their mother."

"You're not able to take care of them right now. We need to get you into rehab and get your life back on track. Then they could come home to you."

Yola jumped to her feet. "No," she screamed. "I'll kill anyone that tries to take them away from me. That includes you or that bitch Ms. Richardson, or the law. Do you understand? Don't you come near us anymore!"

She stormed out of the office, and when Dr. Bridgett made it to the waiting room, it was in time to see the front door swinging closed, the secretary's mouth hanging open in surprise, and nothing in the waiting area but toys and magazines. Yola had taken her children and run.

Ethical Points to Consider:

Mandatory reporting laws for child abuse exist nation-wide. In this case, the children appear to be experiencing neglect because they are often left without an appropriate caregiver. The neglect, and Yola being a flight risk, should be reported to the child protective services caseworker. While this is a mandatory reporting situation, conveying information to protective services is standard procedure in child abuse cases. Therefore, releases of information are signed so that all the counselors, caseworkers, guardians, and agencies involved can communicate regarding the family.

Professionally and ethically, it is important to discuss the possibility of mandated reporting at the outset of therapy with the parent and children (ACA, 2005; APA, 2002; NAADAC, 2008; & NASW, 2008).

If children feel telling the truth in counseling is likely to result in their parents being "in trouble," they are not as likely to be honest. However, in order to more fully protect the children, accurate information is needed. Sometimes information from the children, when investigated, results in their removal from the home. This often disrupts the trust in counseling. Mental health workers report in mandated reporting situations, but they should also take care to explore the trust issues with their clients following mandated reporting. During intake and throughout therapy, the children need to explore the many ways a counselor helps, and the pain associated with therapy. For example, some ways of helping the children's situation improve could include: reporting when necessary, potentially removing the children, etc.

Discussion Questions:

1. What are Yola's key cognitions, emotions, and behaviors that you will integrate into your counseling? Given your identification of these issues, what theoretical orientation would you choose in your work with her? How do you conceptualize the case? What specific techniques and treatment plan would you employ?

2. Does Yola meet the criteria for a diagnosis? If so, what diagnosis(es)?

3. How has her socioeconomic background shaped her cognitive and behavioral choices?

4. How do society's messages about appropriate roles for women impact Yola's life? How will they affect your work with her? How might your own views about drugs, prostitution, and parenting affect your work with her?

5. What is her current potential for suicide? What are the factors that make it more likely? Less likely?

6. Given Yola's threats, what are your opinions regarding warning the Child Protective Services counselor?

7. The children have been in danger previously. What should be done to protect the children from future danger? Or should the workers wait and give Yola a chance to change? How would you help Yola have greater insight into how she puts her children at risk?

8. Yola sees few choices in her life. How would you help her to see broader options?

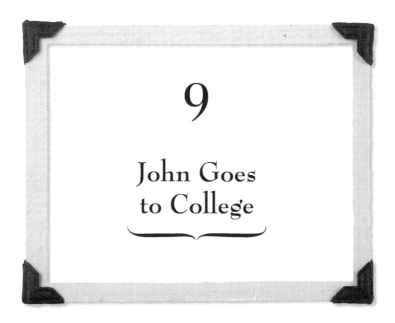

9

John Goes to College

For Your Consideration

As you read about John and his life experiences, be aware of your biases including those surrounding education, opportunities, and potential. Consider whether a diagnosis exists. What would you do if you were John or his parents? What ethical and legal issues are critical?

John's Story

Before high school graduation

John Anderson rolled a can of warm soda between his fingers and sank deeper into the overstuffed sofa in his living room. Empty food containers sat in front of him on the coffee table. He'd spent two days watching news coverage about the Virginia Tech shootings. So many dead, he thought. Was any university safe? John snorted. For that matter, was anywhere safe?

Mixed in the pile of empty sacks and cans sat an opened letter. It was his acceptance to a university in Phoenix. He picked the letter up with shaking fingers and wondered for the hundredth time in the last two days if he should leave his rural community to go to a university darned near the size of his whole town of 40,000. And to top it off, it was surrounded by a million and a half people. John shuddered at the images of so many students packed into a few acres of land, surrounded by overcrowding and traffic and crime. Maybe he shouldn't go. It might be safer to stay right here and go to the local community college.

John sighed. He had to go. His mother was a teacher and she wanted to see him excel in his education. He chewed on his lower lip, deep in thought. *I do love math and art. If I go to Phoenix, maybe I can find a way to use both, like architecture or something.*

Grabbing the remote control, John suddenly shut off the television and got to his feet. He wasn't going to quit. He'd go on to the university and just pay attention to the other students around him. Somebody should have seen the Virginia Tech shooting coming, and he didn't intend to let something like that sneak up on him.

Thanksgiving, freshman year at the university

John sat in freshman comp, ENG101, staring at his essay. Another F. How is it humanly possible to be such a screw up? All of a sudden he was back to reality and heard Dr. Price calling his name, just as the professor released his class for the day.

"Earth to John, John. Good, I see you are back with us. Will you stay after class for a minute?"

John swallowed hard, wondered what was up with the prof, but he walked up front anyway.

"John, thanks for staying. I'm concerned about your grades. In class discussions, I can see you understand the material, but your essays don't show it. Tell me how you write them."

"Well, I sit outside, usually, and sketch out an outline. Then in the library on the computers, I write it out from my ideas and save it."

"Do you write quickly?"

"No, at least it seems slow to me."

"Do you have a chance to edit?"

"Yeah, but I get busy and don't always finish."

"Busy? Just studies or do you go out a lot?"

"Rushing the frat keeps me busy, but if I stay out of the dorm and frat house, I can get my work done at the library and not be bothered with interruptions."

"John, this is your first year at the university. Why don't you go to counseling services and see if they can help you with some coping skills or information, so you can maximize your ability?"

John shrugged. "Thanks, Dr. Price. I'll think about it."

John waited in the small area packed with chairs and comfort-able looking sofas. A variety of students lingered in the room, waiting for appointments with counselors, he supposed. He wasn't doing well at school and had come here for help. John wasn't sure anyone could help, but this was the best he could do. In his hand was a crumpled paper. He'd run his grade averages and was only passing one course out of four. How on earth could he tell his mother that? He forced out a disgusted sigh. What the hell's the matter with me? he wondered.

A pretty young student walked into the waiting area. "John Anderson?"

He bolted to his feet. Surely the counselors weren't this young. She looks about sixteen, he thought. How could he tell her his problems?

She must have seen the shocked expression. "I'm Nancy, the receptionist. Ms. Summers will see you in here." She led the way down a long hall and into a small office, handing over a file with the bazillion papers he had filled out inside.

The middle-aged counselor stood and offered her hand and a ready smile. "John? Have a seat. Let's chat a bit." They sat down and she flipped through the papers. Most were started but not finished. Questions were skipped, answers left blank.

"Tell me what I can help you with, John."

He shrugged. "Don't know really, maybe you can't."

"Let me figure that part out. Fill me in and then perhaps we can put a plan together." She leaned back in her desk chair and waited. The silence grew, pulsed, before John spoke. Then he did so in a rush.

"I'm failing school. My mom's gonna be real disappointed. I can't seem to do anything right. I —"

"Whoa." Ms. Summers chuckled and held up a hand. "You don't have to pour it all out at once. Take a deep breath and tell me what is bothering you."

The young man shook his head, dejected and obviously troubled. "Let's start with some history. Is that okay with you, John?"

"Sure."

He seemed relieved to have some direction.

"Tell me about your physical health."

"Like what? I'm 20 years old, healthy, run at the track when I can find the time. Probably don't eat real well, but that's college life isn't it?"

"It sure can be. What about past history? Surgeries, major illnesses as a child?"

"No surgery. Some illnesses. Typical kid stuff, I suppose."

"Do you remember fevers, things like that?"

"Oh yeah, but I thought most kids did that. I had ear aches a lot and ran a fever with those." He got quiet, seeming to look back into his childhood. "There were a couple times I remember Mom being really worried 'cause I hit higher than 104." He shrugged. "She seemed to think that was bad and got real nervous when that happened."

"What about accidents?"

"Oh, now you are gonna see what a total klutz I am. I broke both arms running out in front of a car once, and another time broke one when I jumped off my bike when it went too fast down a hill."

"Ouch. Anything else? What about your childhood? Do you remember your parents saying when you starting talking and things like that?"

"Just my mom. My dad was never in the picture."

"Do you have brothers and sisters?"

"Two sisters and a brother. They were always lookin' out for me 'cause I was the youngest." He laughed self-consciously. "They said I didn't really do anything much but grunt and point until I went to school. Up until then, they let Mom know what I needed, so I didn't have to say much. But I did start grunting and pointing early, like seven months or something. Does that count?"

"That counts. Thanks for the info, John." She jotted notes on a pad, and then glanced back at him. "How's the social life here at university?"

Another careless shrug. "Oh, you know. Frat parties and stuff."

"Do you enjoy those?"

"To be honest, I feel like they think I'm the country cousin come to town. I put my foot in my mouth sometimes. Kind of make people mad without meaning to, so I usually leave early."

"What about a girl?"

"I have one back home. I miss her, but we both got accepted at different universities."

"Why don't you tell me about her."

John smiled. "Her name is Clara. She's beautiful, but more than that she has a great sense of humor. She is really kind, too. She understands me and my concerns. She always makes me feel better when I'm stressed."

"Any special memories?"

"I'll never forget going to prom. She was like a model in her blue dress, so beautiful. We went to dinner with friends at a fancy country club. Then on to the dance. It was perfect. After the dance, we went to an after party at David's house. We had breakfast and hung out till about 4 a.m. Then I took her home."

His voice trailed off. "Tell me more," Ms. Summers said gently.

"It was so hard to say goodbye and go to different schools. I worry she will meet someone else. I think she is the girl I want to marry. But then I think how smart she is and I'm not. I don't know how to keep her."

"Is there anyone here?"

"I meet girls at the frat parties, but nobody serious."

"John, you indicated here that in middle and high school you got mostly B's and C's. What do you think changed for you here?"

"I don't know. Things just got worse after I graduated high school. That really is pis . . . sorry." He looked sheepish. "It's making me mad. I just can't seem to do as well as I used to. I know I'm smarter than the grades say I am."

"Switching to a major university from high school can be a big change, but I think you're right about how smart you are. What got worse here?"

"I don't know. Just stuff."

Ms. Summers looked at John's graduation date. Not three months after the Virginia Tech shootings. "John, do you think much about Virginia Tech. About those students who died that day?"

"Some," he admitted. "It's just hard to imagine that something like that could happen. All those innocent people just trying to get an education, do better in their lives." John shook his head. "How does that happen?"

"Does it worry you that it could happen here?"

He looked thoughtful for a moment, and she simply waited for his answer. Finally, he spoke. "It could happen anywhere. I know that. Look at all the high school and college shootings going on around the country. Virginia Tech proved it's not safe anywhere anymore."

"What did you think about it?"

"It made me afraid to go to college. I didn't sleep well when I first got here and worried about who my assigned roommate would be. How could they not know what was going to happen? How could the school not stop it? Don't they care about students? I really think about bringing a gun to class sometimes or a taser. Anyway, I just can't think about it."

"You asked about grades," John continued. "Sometimes if students get really low grades, I hear them griping about the professor. Then I worry about what they might do."

"Do you think you are focusing more on the worry than your school work?"

"I don't think so."

"John, I think, from our time together and your former grades, that we should do an evaluation. It's just a few tests that you take and they will give us more information to get to the bottom of this. Would that be all right with you?"

"Sure. That's why I came. I want answers."

They both rose and shook hands. Ms. Summers smiled at him. "Let's set them up for before you go home for Thanksgiving, and we can meet after the break."

December, Freshman Year

"Man, Ms. Summers. I don't know what set my mom off, but she was real defensive about me takin' those tests."

"Did you explain to her what we were doing?"

"I told her it was just to give us a starting point." He shook his head. "I have no idea why she was mad about it."

Ms. Summers opened John's file. She slipped a paper out and turned it toward him so he could read it. John scanned the paper: Full Scale IQ Score 127 with ten points lower on Verbal versus Performance; Wide Range Achievement Test: Reading 55, Spelling 113, Arithmetic 117.

He handed the paper back to her looking more confused than ever. "I hope that means something to you, 'cause it sure doesn't to me."

"Let's talk about them."

An hour after John left, Nancy buzzed her intercom. "Ms. Summers, there's a Mrs. Anderson on line three. Do you want me to take a message?"

"No, thanks. I'll take it." She figured she might as well get this one over with and not save it for later.

"Ms. Summers here. May I help you?"

"This is Mrs. Anderson. I'm John Anderson's mother. I want to know what is going on with my son."

"Have you spoken to him about that?"

"I have and he said you did some tests. What were they and what are you looking for? I demand to know what is wrong with my son."

Ms. Summers rubbed her suddenly throbbing temple. She hated these calls.

"Are you going to answer me, Ms. Summers? I have a right to know about my child's well-being."

The question was a demand indeed. Ms. Summers took a deep breath and spoke to Mrs. Anderson as calmly as possible, trying to reassure the woman she knew was only worried about her son.

Ethical Points to Consider:

In this case, we find a college student who has reached the age to consent to treatment. Colleges often face navigating between students consenting to treatment and their privacy rights, as opposed to their parents who are paying the college bills and want information regarding their "children." According to Remley and Herlihy (2007), the parents of students in college can receive student records without student's consent, if the student was claimed on the parent's taxes. However, Reley and Herlihy point out that this law does not apply to records maintained by the mental health worker. That is, parental review of college academic records would not include case notes that are maintained by the mental health worker (Remley & Herlihy).

Support offices for students with disabilities at colleges and universities are very cautious regarding to whom information is released. Faculty are notified that a student qualifies as having a disability and what appropriate accommodations are, but not the nature of the disability. For example, a student might present their professor with a letter indicating he/she has a qualifying disability and that extended testing time in a private room is appropriate. However, the professor is not informed about the specifics, such as the student having a learning disability or psychiatric disorder. This is to protect the student's privacy.

Within public school settings, school counselors face similar situations with students who are tested and diagnosed. Even with appropriate releases, they must balance the needs for teachers to have enough information to assist the student without providing unnecessary and excessive information that violates the student's right to privacy.

Discussion Questions:

1. What are John's significant cognitions, emotions, and behaviors? Given your identification of these, what diagnosis(es) might be appropriate?

2. Based on the issues you have identified and any diagnoses, what theoretical orientation will guide your work with him? What is your conceptualization of the treatment plan?

3. How do cultural and developmental factors impact how you visualize treatment for John?

4. How does the recent violence at universities impact John and his concerns?

5. What information should be given to his mother, and how should she be integrated into treatment or excluded from treatment?

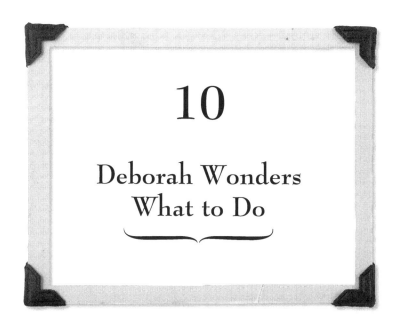

10

Deborah Wonders What to Do

For your consideration

As you read about Deborah, consider not only her circumstances, but those of people surrounding her. How does the environment impact her and exacerbate or improve her symptoms?

Deborah's Story

Monday, April 9

Deborah ignored Karen's scowl and kept cooking supper, even though there were regulations against cooking in the dorms.

"Deborah, you're going to get us in so much trouble. You can't do that up here."

"I have to eat," she snapped. "The food isn't safe in the student union. It's all spoiled."

Karen sighed. "You know hundreds of students eat there every day and don't get sick."

"I don't know that. What happens to them when they go back to their rooms? Besides those people are just after me, not the others."

"Those people?"

"Yes. The ones down there in the cafeteria. And my teachers, too." She whispered the last as though hiding from conspiracy.

Karen surrendered and sniffed the air. "Mexican tonight?"

"Tacos. I made plenty if you want some. This new hot plate works really well."

"Okay. If we get caught cooking we're both in trouble, so I may as well make it worth it."

The two girls ate in silence, then Karen wiped her mouth with a paper towel. "Uh, Deborah, do you think you ought to talk to someone about these people who are out to get you? If the professors are really doctoring your grades, you need to file a complaint."

"I appreciate it, Karen, but the truth is no one will believe me."

"Have you been in class? Can't you talk to them?"

Deborah shrugged carelessly. "I didn't go this week. Maybe next week."

"You have to go or you're going to fail for sure. What will your folks say then?"

"They won't like it, but I have to protect myself."

"Don't they pick up the tab for your education and housing?"

"Sure. They can afford it."

"Affording it and throwing money away if you aren't in class are two different things."

Trying to change the subject, Deborah asked, "Are you going by Ted's tonight after class?"

Karen smiled. "Yep. I won't be back tonight."

"Okay. I'll block the door, so if you change your mind, call me so I can let you in."

"All right." She got to her feet dusting crumbs off her jeans. "Thanks for the tacos." She set her plate aside. "See you."

Deborah watched the door close behind her roommate. She was on her own for the night. All she had to do was burn the lights all night and put a chair under the door handle. She'd be safe until morning.

Deborah missed class the rest of the week, afraid to go into the rooms with other students and the professors. Whenever she thought about eating at the student union she remembered the food was dangerous and meant to hurt her. She'd end up cooking grilled cheese or soup in the room. Besides, she hated being in the crowds of students. The boys always watched her, staring, and thinking about ways to hurt her. Now even the girls were doing it. She couldn't stand being where they could all point and talk, making plans to harm her in some way. Maybe they were the ones paying the cafeteria people to serve her spoiled food.

Then she knew, the food *was* meant to hurt all of them. The other students didn't deserve to be hurt any more than she did.

Hurrying from the crowded room, Deborah glanced around furtively, watching for any move toward her that was threatening in any way. She scurried down the sidewalk, up to her room, and slammed the door, leaning back against it and breathing as though the demons of hell had been chasing her.

Friday, April 13

Deborah knew this was the day that all the students were going to be poisoned. She raced out of the dorm, across campus, and into the front of the student union. She stood in the main entrance where most students entered. She couldn't cover all the doors, but maybe she could get some of the others to cover smaller entrances.

She didn't recognize anyone, so just started calling out, "Go down the street to the village to eat. The food is poisoned here." She grabbed at students' sleeves as they tried to pass, imploring them to do as she asked.

"Please, please don't eat here. You'll die."

She saw the shocked expressions and the obvious desire of her fellow students to get away from her. Maybe they were part of the plan against her. No, she reasoned, they were in danger, too. She had to spirit them away from here.

It didn't take long for a campus cop to show up. "Miss, you need to leave and go on home now." He seemed concerned to Deborah.

"Officer, these people are trying to poison all the students. You have to help me stop them from going in the dining areas."

"Well, now it isn't the best food —"

"No! You don't understand. They are trying to kill us."

"Who is?" he asked.

"All of them, everyone in here. They're trying to kill all of us, especially me because I'm trying to stop them."

"All right, then. I'll get some help for us." He pressed the radio on his shoulder. "This is Johnson. I need an ambulance at the student union. We've got a student in crisis over here."

"Right away. Stay put."

"Oh, I will," he said, turning back to try and keep her talking so she'd stop calling out to the others.

Deborah swung toward the front doors when she heard sirens. Were they there to help her or were they part of it, too? she wondered.

"It's all right, young lady. They're here to help you."

He seemed to have guessed at her suspicions. But his voice was kind. Could she trust him?

Deborah woke up in the psychiatric ward of St. Michael's Hospital. Her parents stood at her bedside. As usual, her father wore a grimacing frown and her mother wrung her hands as tears slipped down her cheeks. They whispered as though Deborah couldn't hear them. Did they think she was in a coma, for God's sake?

"If you have something to say, say it," Deborah snapped. "I have to get out of here. They are going to kill me if I don't get away." She tried to sit up but fell back against the pillow as her vision blurred. They told her she'd been medicated in the ambulance, but she didn't remember any of it. What did they give me? she wondered. There isn't anything wrong with me. This is just more of them trying to hurt me. She glanced quickly around the room. I have to get out of here. How can I?

"Get me out of here," she snarled. "I'm your daughter. You have to help me."

Her mother looked away, muttering that Deborah wasn't their little girl, not the girl she had born and raised to have an important part in society. "How could this happen? Where did we fail her, Charles?"

Her father simply shook his head still frowning and offering no comfort to Deborah at all. "I don't know Martha, but it's obvious she isn't our girl anymore or she wouldn't do this."

"It's not me! Don't you get it? They're trying to kill me! What am I going to do?"

"We can't help you anymore. The doctors will do it. Goodbye, Deborah." He took Martha by the elbow, turned her away and Deborah watched them leave, her mother stifling a sob.

Now what? They'd abandoned her to her fate. How can I get away? She tried to sit again as the questions fired at her fast, tripping over one another. One thing she knew for sure: if she didn't get away, they'd kill her. Hopeless, she fell back against the pillow for a second time.

Dr. Martin came into her room, attempting to squelch the rage he felt. He had just finished speaking to her parents and learned they were cutting her off because of her college performance and her "illness." "More money than brains," he muttered. Hadn't he explained she hadn't dropped out because she wanted to? That she had serious medical issues to deal with? They could pay for the best for this girl, help her through this, and instead they were protecting themselves from what they thought would be embarrassing and denying any liability to leave her in the county ward. She had not renewed her student medical insurance, so she had none. He looked at the frightened young woman and wondered how some parents slept at night. At least he found out from them she wasn't like this prior to college. There were no significant medical or mental health issues in her history.

"Deborah, I'm Dr. Martin. How are you feeling?"

She looked terrified and sank back against her pillow. She didn't answer.

"I'm here to help you, Deborah. Why don't you tell me what happened yesterday?"

"Nothing happened," she snapped. "They're trying to kill me. You have to help me get away if you're really here to help."

"Why don't we get acquainted and then I can help you better?"

She looked him up and down, and seemed to be assessing his trustworthiness.

"Okay," she said finally. "What do you want to know?"

"Tell me about school. How's that been for you, Deborah?"

"All right, until this last semester. The professors are trying to flunk me." Her voice had dropped to a conspiratorial level. "They want to get rid of me."

"Why would they do that?"

"They don't like me, don't want me there."

"Why, Deborah?"

A tear rolled down her cheek then. "I don't know. Nobody ever likes me. They all want me to go away. I got fired four different times."

"What were you doing? Job wise, I mean."

"Not much. I worked as an office clerk, but they fired me because I wouldn't let some dangerous looking people come inside. I sent them away."

"Then what did you do?" He jotted notes down as she spoke.

"I was a waitress in the village. But they didn't like me either."

"What happened there?"

Now she sounded angry. "All I did was try to protect their patrons. I'd seat them at one table, then when I realized it wasn't safe I moved them to another. Mostly they thought I was moving them to a better table. Then for a while I had to move them during their meals. They didn't like that. They started complaining. So they fired me."

Dr. Martin noted Deborah's quick glances around the room. She watched everything, seemed afraid of every shadow, every sound. "Deborah, can you tell me if you hear voices in your mind?"

Deborah laughed and quickly looked side-to-side around the room. "Of course not. That would make me crazy, wouldn't it?"

"Not crazy, just in need of some help straightening things out."

Deborah threw her blanket aside and crawled out of bed. She paced back and forth, then moved to the small closet. "I'm not crazy. You're making things up. Why are you doing this to me?" She opened and slammed doors.

"Where are my clothes? I want to get out of here." She was screaming now. "You're one of them," she said backing away from him as he tried to reach her.

"No, I'm not. I want to help you." He thought of the level of disturbance his young patient felt and knew this wasn't his field of expertise. She needed a specialist, but how could he refer her when she had no insurance, no money.

"Deborah, come on back and sit down. I won't hurt you." He only wanted to help, but he only worked at county one day a week. He decided he would do the best he could for her, since they had no referral options.

Dr. Martin thought to himself that this girl was going to need a long course of treatment.

It was two weeks before Deborah was able to go home. Her roommate, Karen, picked her up at the hospital and took her back to their dorm room. She offered to drive her to see Dr. Martin at his office for her appointment the following day.

"Thanks, Karen." Deborah was subdued, taking medication that made her feel lethargic, but at least she felt calmer. She didn't seem able to focus, though, and knew she'd have to leave the dorm soon and find a place to stay. But, she wondered, how could she find a safe place to live with no money of her own? Her parents wouldn't answer her calls that just proved they were out to get her, too.

Deborah walked into Dr. Martin's office and took a seat. He smiled at her and tried to reassure her that she was safe in his office.

"I'm so glad you came to see me. How was it to be back at school yesterday?"

Deborah shrugged. "Okay, I guess. I'm not in class anymore, but I don't need it anyway."

"Why is that, Deborah?"

"I already have a job lined up at the Museum of Art."

She glanced around the room, and he noted she had carefully chosen a chair that allowed her to keep her back to the wall and an eye on the door.

"What will you be doing?" He'd been trained to not lay out expectations, but he was surprised by her answer.

"I'm an expert on art history, so I'll be authenticating pieces of art," she said it nonchalantly, like everyone should know her and know her work. Her authority was not to be questioned.

Dr. Martin cleared his throat. Thought a minute. "Is that what you were studying in college?"

"No. Well, I did take two classes, but English was my major."

"Where did you learn about art history?" Her family has money, he thought, perhaps she'd traveled extensively.

"Oh, I don't know. I've just always known about it. Now I'm a respected expert in the field."

He gazed at his patient. Nice young woman, he thought, but she makes no sense.

"Have you spoken to your parents lately?"

"No. They won't take my calls. I have no idea what's the matter with them. I went to college just like they wanted, now I have an important job waiting for me. They just don't get it."

"Don't get what, Deborah?"

"How special I am. I need to be protected. I can't let anyone get me. I have important work to do."

"What are the voices saying?"

Her demeanor changed in a flash. "I told you at the hospital, I don't hear voices. Nobody listens to me." She clasped her hands in her lap, glancing constantly about the room and at the door.

He waited out the silence. Then Deborah whispered, "They warn me about the poisoned food. Don't trust the cooks. I try to warn people but more and more people are trying to trick me."

"All right, Deborah. I think we can work together to turn down the volume on the voices." Dr. Martin wished for the tenth time Deborah had the resources to be referred to a specialist. He shook his head. All he could do was his best and hope it was enough.

Ethical Points to Consider:

The psychologist who saw this client on an in-patient basis is trying to refer her for treatment. Her lack of insurance and financial resources are a problem. While at some point she may receive social security disability, currently she does not. Referral and advocacy on the part of this client to appropriate social support agencies is critical. In terms of fees, Remley and Herlihy (2007) point out that any sliding scale fees must be consistent across clients, irrespective of having insurance and not based on the client being a member of a protected category. Ethical codes (ACA, 2005; & APA, 2002) require notifying clients if the use of bill collection agencies could occur. Additionally, when clients are unable to pay fees, ethical codes require referral to other agencies rather than abandoning the client (ACA, 2005; & APA, 2002). Recommending pro bono work, or work performed for little or no pay is common in professional codes of ethics. Mental health professionals are expected to "give back" to their communities professionally. Many do this via work with disaster relief, homeless shelters, and other similar agencies.

Another way is to counsel some clients for free. However, there are potential difficulties with this. The mental health professional needs to consider how many sessions to offer for free, with clear criteria regarding which clients receive free sessions. (Remley & Herlihy, 2007)

Discussion Questions:

1. What are Deborah's key cognitions, emotions, and behaviors that you will integrate into your counseling? Given your identification of these issues, what theoretical orientation would you choose in your work with her? How do you conceptualize the case? What specific techniques and treatment plan would you employ?

2. Does Deborah have a mental disorder(s)? If so, what? What is her global assessment of functioning score at the beginning of the week, upon admission, and at her follow-up outpatient appointment?

3. How has her socioeconomic background and university setting shaped her cognitive and behavioral choices?

4. How do societal expectations for behavior in a dorm and university setting impact Deborah?

5. Is Deborah at risk for suicide? What factors make it more likely? Less likely?

6. What strengths or assets does Deborah have that you will build on in your counseling?

7. What is your opinion of Dr. Martin's idea to offer pro bono therapy? If it appears there may be competency issues, what do you recommend?

8. In your place of residence, can medication be mandated? Would you suggest Deborah be put on mandated medication if she refused voluntary compliance? Why or why not?

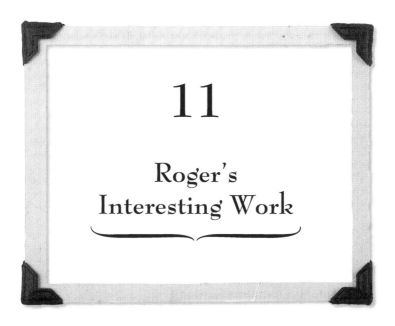

11

Roger's Interesting Work

For Your Consideration

As you read about Roger and his experiences, be aware of your biases and how they impact your interpretation of the case. Where is the line between motivation, entrepreneurship, and dysfunction? Various options exist from different theoretical perspectives. Consider which, if any, you would recommend.

Roger's Story

Day 1

Roger Schwartzbein snapped his cell phone shut, smiling smugly. Another sale. What a great week this is, he thought. Ninety high-end shoe sales in five days. Not bad. Roger snorted. His wife had tackled him that morning, complaining about him not getting enough sleep. *I don't need sleep, not when I can work.*

The way he saw it, there was no point in wasting time sleeping when he could be productive instead. He was building a scheme in his head, a way to make a lot of money fast. He didn't want to waste a minute.

With that thought in mind, he glanced across the lot as a nice Buick parked and a suited businessman stepped out. Roger looked at the shoe store where he worked and saw several other sales people coming out. Better get with it, Roger, or you'll lose the sale to someone else.

Day 2

"Damn it, Ken. I'm telling you Roger stole a customer right out from under me," Patricia complained.

"I'm sure he didn't do it intentionally," their manager intoned.

"Yes, he did." She said it slowly, deliberately letting each word settle on the boss. Patricia knew Roger brought in more sales, and consequently more money, than anyone else in the store. That meant the manager would side with him no matter what. But hadn't Roger's sales slipped in the last couple of weeks? He couldn't finish the sales, moving on to steal customers from other sales people, rather than finishing up his own sales.

"Do you want sales people you can't trust in here, Ken? People that would stab you in the back in a heartbeat if they thought they could steal this entire company away from you?"

Ken had the good graces to look embarrassed when he shook his head. "I'm sure he wouldn't do that, or steal your customers."

"I'm not the only one he's screwed. Talk to some of the others." She got to her feet, pacing back and forth in front of the massive mahogany desk. "You might be surprised if you check into some of his dealings. They are less than appropriate." She stalked out of Ken's office, letting the door slam shut. Let him think about that. In the meantime, she intended to have a word with Roger.

She found him in his corner office, one she knew well and used to occupy, until he'd become the high seller. It was all glass windows and looked out over Veterans Park. The thought of the green expanse of lawn outside the windows giving way to flowers, fountains, and trees should have comforted her, but they didn't. All she wanted was to strangle Roger. She stopped in front of the heavy wood door, thumping unceremoniously on the carved design.

"Come on in."

He sounded friendly, trustworthy. More like a viper, she thought. When she walked in, she found him with a huge smile plastered on his face. She could wipe that off his lips; she knew it.

She stopped in front of him, placed her fists on her hips.

"What the hell do you mean taking that woman? She was mine."

He shrugged innocently. "I wasn't aware anyone had been working with her on the wedding order. She didn't say anything."

"You know damn well I had been showing her the shoes last week."

"That may be, but you weren't around when she needed you yesterday, so I offered to help her."

"You can't keep this up, Roger."

"I can do anything I want." He stood and rose to his full height. "I can do exactly what I like. I have Ken in the palm of my hand. I'm making sales left and right. You don't stand a chance against me. If you aren't happy with the smaller sales I leave you, get out."

She looked into his eyes and saw wildness there — kind of a power or infallibility somehow. She knew he was beyond listening. Turning, she walked out the door and back toward her office, making plans to look for a more reputable place to work.

Roger watched her go and shook his head. Sore loser, he thought. She can't stand a little honest competition from a master. He grinned and sat again, lifting his phone to make more calls.

Day 3

Roger walked into First State Bank, straight to the loan manager's desk. She had her head bent over the papers there and jumped when he spoke to her.

"Lori, how are you?" His voice was soft, warm and seductive. The image of his wife flew across his mind's eye, but any guilt he might have felt quickly slid away. This was pure business. "How's it going? Have I got a deal for you."

"Fine, Roger." A light blush spread over her cheeks. "Nice to see you again. Can I help you?"

He smiled and sat across from her, lifting his briefcase onto the flat surface of her desk. "I want to get a pre-approval to purchase several hundred high-end shoes."

She frowned and, he thought, looked a bit disappointed. Was she expecting something more personal? he wondered.

"What kind of business?"

"Well, don't tell anyone, but I know I can trust you, honey. Here's the deal, I am buying the shoes at a factory reject store and reselling them at the shoe store where I work. I can make more money on them."

She gave a low whistle. "That sounds pretty risky. How do you think you can sell them over there? Won't they have to be sold as rejects?"

Roger huffed out a breath. Another person telling him his ideas wouldn't work. No one seemed to have any foresight but him. "I'm buying the ones in good shape that look good, and turning them around so fast there's no inventory cost. It's not like I have to register them. I am going to make a lot of money off each one by selling them just under suggested retail for new."

"Well, if you're sure . . . Okay, we can do that."

She sounded disappointed that they were only talking business and pleasure filled him at the response a mere refusal of his company brought to her. She was so easy, not even a challenge.

"I'd appreciate it. Perhaps we can get the paper work done, and then we could go out and celebrate over dinner. Would you like that?"

"We're not really supposed to go out with clients, but it does sound lovely. Aren't you expected at home?"

"That can wait."

She continued typing, bringing up new screens on her computer. "You look happy. Business must be good since I saw you last."

"I'm on top of the world. Nothing can stop me now. After the shoes sell, I'm using the profits on motor homes. I'll turn those over, too. I can sell anything"

"We need some new information on you," she said. "It's been a while and the financials will need to be updated."

He pulled his sales figures from the case and arrogantly tossed them on the desk in front of her. "They can't question the loan. I've made enough this month to pay cash for it, but I don't want to wait for our end of month commissions to come in."

"All right, Roger. Let's have a look."

When he left the bank, Roger knew nothing could take him down. He was on an upward climb that no one could stop. He hit the fast dial for his home. "Hey, Babe," he said when his wife answered. "How you doin?"

"I'm fine. Where are you?"

She sounded suspicious, but he ignored it. Nothing was going to bring his mood down — nothing. "Hey Sweet Thing, I have to work late. I'm working on the new plan I told you about."

"Roger, don't you think we should talk more about that? It's a lot of money. Can we afford to risk it?"

"It's not a risk," he snapped, suddenly angry. "Trust me, damn it. I know what I'm doing." He had reached his vehicle and opened the door to drop his briefcase on the seat.

"I do trust you, I just think —"

"Don't think and don't worry. I have it all under control. See you tomorrow."

He snapped the cell closed and slid it into his suit jacket pocket. He hurried into the SUV and headed for the shoe outlet. He had things to do.

Later, Roger pulled into The Smoke House Restaurant. One valet opened the door for Lori, and another came around to open his door.

After climbing out, Roger took her hand and led her through the front doors. They were celebrating the deal that would net him a small fortune. He could move on and stop selling ordinary shoes. He had big plans for tonight, too. A nice dinner, good wine, and a night in the best room at the Double Door Inn. Everything in his future looked bright.

And tonight he'd spend in the arms of one hot, sexy woman. Roger smiled. It couldn't get much better than this.

Day 4

"But Ken, think about it. This is a win-win for both of us."

"How do you figure?" Ken rocked back in his chair rocking slightly as he often did when stressed.

"I paid for the shoes, so no money out of your pocket. I'll be advertising them, so no cost to you. When I sell them, you get a commission, money in your pocket. It can't get better than that."

"Technically, you know we can't sell any shoes as new from the factory except the first quality ones we purchase from the company. How are we supposed to account for these shoes?"

"I know a way. All we have to do is show them as used to the company, but sell them as new."

Ken rocked harder. "Roger, that is very close to crossing an ethical line, maybe even a legal one. I'm not sure about this."

"Lighten up." Roger jumped to his feet and began pacing.

"We can both make a pile of money in spite of the rotten economy. I tell you, it will work. Just have some faith in me. I can do this."

A heavy silence filled the room. One beat, two . . .

"Ken, I'm the best salesman you have. I can go anywhere else in the city and get a job today." He shrugged nonchalantly.

"I don't want to leave here, but I've purchased these shoes. I'll leave if I have to, in order to make this deal."

"I don't like threats." Ken got up now and leaned across his desk toward Roger.

His tone friendly, Roger said, "It's not a threat, Ken, just a fact. I want this deal. I'd like to make us both a pile of money."

Ken dropped onto his chair. "All right," he said with a shake of his head. "Let's hope we don't lose our jobs in the process."

Roger strode into his own office and stood in front of the glass expanse that looked over the city park. Why didn't anybody trust him? Didn't they know he was good, probably the best. His good mood threatened to vanish, but then he saw a customer pull onto the lot in a high-end Cadillac. Maybe they need pricey shoes to push the gas pedal, he thought, heading for his door to beat his colleagues to the punch. They could sell the small, cheap shoes. The big fish were his.

Jonathan walked out of the side door of the store a step ahead of him, but Roger quickly skirted him and called out a greeting to the couple getting out of the baby blue Caddy.

Apparently having had too much of Roger, Jonathan grabbed his arm, jerking him to a stop and swinging him around.

"We're all getting damn tired of you stealing all the customers."

Roger smiled. "I can't help it if you don't get to them quick enough. I'm on the ball, that's all."

"No, you're not. You're an unethical jerk and the sooner Ken realizes that, the better."

Seeing the confrontation, the elderly couple glanced at each other and scurried back to their car, quickly pulling out of the lot.

Roger's smile disappeared. "See what the hell you did," he screamed. "Those people looked like hot ones and you scared them off." Roger shoved Jonathan nearly knocking him down.

"Keep your hands off me." He shoved Roger back. "You won't listen to anyone. You and your crazy schemes. You can't sell those shoes anyway, but as second quality, which means you can't get anything for them close to retail. You're going to lose your shirt on that deal. And it serves you right." He turned to leave, but Roger hauled him back around.

"You sorry son-of-a-bitch. I know what I'm doing," he screamed. "You can't stand it because I'm better than you." He took a swing at Jonathan who easily ducked the punch.

"What the hell's the matter with you? Knock it off."

Ken and several salespeople ran from the store to break up the two men. Jonathan was continuing to duck Roger's flailing fists.

Roger's balance seemed off as he swung around to watch the others running toward them, fear showing in his eyes. He called out to them to stop, but his voice slurred and he didn't recognize his own words.

Ken held up his hands in a placating gesture. "Take it easy, Roger. Everything's okay." Under his breath he said to Jonathan, "Go call 9-1-1. Something's not right here."

Roger started yelling, "You can't handle a great salesman. I'm selling these shoes down at the Double Door. Where is Lori when I need her? I need to sign the forms, what a great day. Hey, let's go to the park and shoot some hoops. Get your hands off my shoes."

Roger glanced up as a man stepped into the room, flip chart in hand. The little twerp had a smile plastered on his face Roger knew was false.

The man looked up from the chart. "Mr. Schwartzbein, I'm Bill Littleton. How are you doing?"

"How do you think?" Roger snapped. "I have to get out of here and back to work." He frowned at the doctor. "I have deals to make. A family to take care of. I have to move fast. Losing time. Losing money. I have to get out of here. You're holding me back. Gonna be great!"

Littleton ignored his non-stop ranting that made no sense. "Have you had any episodes like this before?"

"No. I'm fine. I don't belong in here with these fruitcakes. Get me out of here. You ever been to the Double Door? Let's go get a drink and meet some ladies."

"Mr. Schwartzbein, I can't help you if you don't cooperate."

"I don't have to. I want to be released right now!"

"I'm sorry. You're being kept for 72-hour observation. If you help me, we might be able to get you out after that."

"You can't force me to stay. I have shoes to sell. Money to make. Don't you know anything? Get me Lori and Cynthia and I need a phone. NOW!"

"I'll know more if you talk to me." Bill shut the chart.

Roger kept going on about some shoes. It made no sense.

"Look, Roger, I'm sorry this happened to you, but you can't leave until we figure out what's going on." Bill scanned the man's features and saw stress and anger there. Obviously he'd been counting on this deal. Roger's wife had told him that he had used their home as collateral for a huge loan. "I've been needing some good shoes. When we get you back on your feet and feeling better, how about I come look at the shoes?"

Roger's mood seemed to lift a bit. "Sure," he said sliding into salesman mode. "What style?"

156

Bill stepped into the hall and walked up to Roger's wife, Cynthia. "Mrs. Schwartzbein, he's settling down a bit now. Can you tell me some more of the history?"

She nodded and then sipped from a cup of coffee. Bill gently took her elbow, turned her away from the room and led her to a row of chairs along the wall.

"How's Roger been sleeping?"

Cynthia shook her head. "He doesn't, at least not much. He brags he only needs two hours of sleep a night." She huffed out a little breath. "He claims that is when he is most creative and comes up with all his ideas."

"What does he do the rest of the night? He can't be working very effectively then."

"I couldn't say, but I'd guess he's having great sex with his lover, the town tramp. I wouldn't know because he isn't at home."

"I'm sorry. Do you know how long this behavior's been going on? Has he had trouble before?"

She shook her head. "The affair started recently. As far as I know he's never been physically or mentally ill."

"Educational history?"

"High school. We met there. He finished and then went to work selling."

"Family other than you?"

"His father's an astronomer. They moved to the desert and away from the city so he could see the sky and avoid the light pollution. He was an only child. I think his dad might have been disappointed he didn't follow his footsteps and go to college to become a professor."

"Well, we'll see what we can do to help him. Are you all right?"

She nodded, then looked at Bill. "We have to get him on his feet and back to his deal. I didn't want him to borrow that money, but he insisted he knew what he was doing. We'll lose everything if he's wrong. We barely survived his last big idea."

Ethical Points to Consider:

In Roger's situation, we find a dilemma often faced by mental health professionals. A client has something we desire. This could be expert knowledge or access to something. For example, a stock broker, financial advisor, tax accountant, realtor, lawyer, medial doctor, salesperson, etc. Our perception that the clients could help us via their advice or getting a "good" deal is very tempting. This is a slippery slope. For instance, is it ok to ask them for a referral to someone in the business? If so, do you mention who sent you? Or, is it ok to go to them after the counseling ends because you trust they will help you get a fair price on a car or house? Perhaps you know they need the money. Ethics codes caution professionals in this area (ACA, 2005; APA, 2002; NAADAC, 2008; & NASW, 2008). It is important to first consider the client's wellbeing. Is it in the client's best interest to help the mental health professional get a good deal on a car or a referral to a tax accountant? The answer is usually "no." The ACA (2005) *Code of Ethics* cautions against any relationships with former clients. Clients often return for additional counseling, sometimes years later. If the counselor has had a personal relationship with the client in the interim, the possibility of serving again as that client's counselor is compromised. Thus, it is best to avoid relationships outside of treatment both during and following counseling.

Discussion Questions:

1. What are Roger's cognitions, emotions, and behaviors? What are the critical issues that need to be addressed? Given your identification of these, what theoretical orientation would you choose in your work with him? How do you conceptualize the case? What specific techniques and treatment plan would you employ?

2. How might his job in sales contribute to the problem or be part of the solution?

3. What, if any, diagnosis(es) would you make? Which symptoms support your decision?

4. Do you agree with placing Roger on a 72-hour hold? Explain your opinion.

5. Assume you live in a location that permits court-mandated medication. What evidence in the case history supports or argues against mandatory medication for Roger?

6. Assume Roger recovers and is fine. Bill was already in the market for dress shoes. What is your opinion about Bill purchasing them at Roger's store, assuming he uses a different sales person?

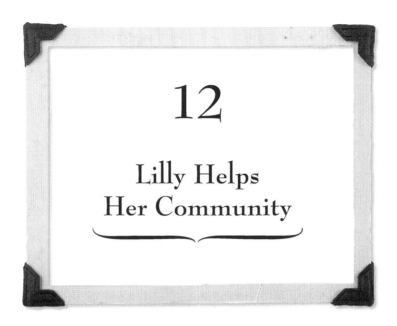

12

Lilly Helps
Her Community

For Your Consideration

As you read the following case, consider the competing demands on Lilly in serving relief workers, survivors, and herself. How would you balance these demands given the events that unfold?

Lilly's Story

Lilly Santiago settled onto the comfortable blue sofa and smiled uneasily at Bill Jorgensen. The room was decorated in the same muted colors as the rest of the psychiatric unit of the hospital, comforting she supposed. Not unlike her office before she retired. Her focus slid back to the man across from her. The blond psychologist was young, and she wondered if he could help someone who'd seen more than he might even be able to imagine. It still rankled her that she was in the hospital — but she knew the fact that she didn't remember being brought here, much less what happened before, and that was why she was here. She knew she was a counselor, had been for years. She should be able to deal with her own stress without seeking professional assistance.

What would you tell a friend to do? her inner voice nudged her. "Shut up," she mumbled.

"Excuse me?" Bill asked as he looked up from his notes.

"Sorry." She gave him a sheepish smile. "Just talking to myself. Think that's a bad sign?"

Bill laughed with her at the old joke, and then focused his gaze on her face. "Why don't you tell me how you got here? I see from your admission papers you're a counselor, too."

"I don't know how I got here. I feel silly, really." She plucked at a full deep orange robe that flowed down around her ankles.

"Why do you feel silly? We all need help once in a while. Tell me about yourself."

"I work with a group called Counselors Providing Relief (CPR). I left for Florida a few days ago and the next thing I know, I'm here."

Bill smiled. "I know about that group. Great bunch of people doing good things."

Lilly shifted in her seat, a bit uncomfortable with the praise even if it was for the entire group and not her. "I thought so. I joined them when I retired from practice a couple of years ago. By the time I turned fifty-three, I'd pretty much seen the same kind of one-on-one clients over and over again. I wanted to help the community in a broader sense."

"And the problem with that is?"

"It's a pretty stressful time when you get sent to a disaster site. You see a lot of bad things," she said quietly with a shrug. "Like this assignment in Florida, water and wind — I knew there would be a lot of damage. A lot of loss. I don't know what happened, but I guess something is wrong, because here I am." She became very tearful.

"Tell me about the tears."

"I just don't know. I want to keep working with CPR." She linked and unlinked her fingers. "To do that, I have to get better. They say I have to come to terms with whatever got me here."

"Have you ever taken a break from the disaster work? Done anything fun to release the tension from the experiences?"

Lilly nodded. "I have, yes. I went to see my family in Central America and traveled to my old home village. That was nice. Maybe I am just stressed now." She knew she didn't sound convinced so why should he be?

"Why don't you begin by telling me what kind of problems you're having that you think are stress related?"

"The usual list, I guess. Sleep disturbances, weight gain. Of course, that is probably menopause." She laughed self-consciously and looked down. "I just cannot remember how I got here and why they won't let me go to the next job."

"I can see why you want to get this taken care of before it goes too far."

Her tears continued to escape and slide down her cheeks. Bill handed her the ever-present counselor's box of tissues. "Thanks," she said with a sniffle.

"Do you remember your last disaster assignment?"

"I remember getting on the plane."

"Lilly, what do you think about hypnosis to help you tell me what happened? It might uncover some subconscious memories so I can better understand. Afterward, together we can uncover the memories consciously, as you are ready for them."

"Okay." She shrugged. "I'll try anything."

"Get comfortable now, Lilly. Lean back and just breathe. Slow and deep. Let your eyes drift closed if you prefer." He waited while she took a few deep breaths, and then continued talking slowly, reassuringly until Lilly slipped into a very relaxed state. Once she was hypnotized, silence filled the room, except for the trickle of water from a bamboo fountain in the corner. "When you're ready, tell me what happened at that site."

With Bill's help, Lilly drifted back, going to Hurricane David in her mind's eye.

Memories during hypnosis

"Lilly, tell me about Florida. Are you there yet?"

"Yes, I see it. Palm trees are swaying in a gentle breeze. It looks almost peaceful, but I know it's not going to be. . . We're landing now. Ooh, it's a narrow landing strip. I'm worried. It took forever for us to get approval that it was safe to go in and help.

"It was like the plane and supplies were wrapped in red tape, like a bird caught in a net, unable to fly until they cut it free."

Lilly shivered and fell silent, her eyelids flickering. Bill shook out a small quilt from the sofa and laid it over her. "It's all right, Lilly. You're safe here. Just see it like a movie. Do not feel the fear or emotions. Just watch it."

"We're ready to leave the airport to go south through the everglades. I don't know if it's safe for the team until the disaster relief has been fully deployed and arrives with provisions and fresh water."

Lilly's words drifted away.

"It's all right, Lilly. You're safe here. You can continue when you're ready. Breathe deep and relax."

She sucked in a soul-deep breath and slowly let it slip between her lips. "Thousands need our help. Loved ones are buried in rubble, lost in the flood waters; houses and all their worldly possessions gone from the force of the wind and high tides. The people who survived need us to get through the coming days as well as possible. We have to go on.

"I am the director of this team, and the safety of my staff as well as our team's effectiveness are on me. So much responsibility. So much to be seen to, supplies to get in, people to counsel."

"Are you off the plane yet?"

"Yes."

Suddenly she spoke as though her team was in front of her. "Come on, everyone. Grab your bags and let's get to work, shall we?"

"They're looking at me. So fresh, so young and new in the field. They probably haven't seen the devastation they're about to experience. Most of these kids will end up needing debriefing and more serious counseling themselves by the time we're done here.

"A man with a disaster relief jacket is waiting on the tarmac. He sees the clipboard in my hand and looks at me. 'Ms. Santiago?' he's asking.

"'That's right. Mr. Whitaker?'

"'Right you are. Call me Charles. We have the trucks over here to take your crew to the shelter area. Will you come with me, please?'

"'Come on folks. Grab your things and get them to the trucks. We're being taken to the relief area.'

"I'm hurrying after Mr. Whitaker with the others trailing us. I look back at the airfield as we walk. Huge felled trees bisect a couple of hangers. Debris is caught on the sea side of the structures. No doubt it blew in with the force of the hurricane."

"How big was the storm, Lilly?"

"A Class IV . . . left little standing close to the sea, and it isn't much better in the inland towns from what I was told. What the floodwaters haven't destroyed, the mud has.

"I see people wandering across the airfield carrying bundles of clothing and bedding. It must be all of their possessions tucked inside the fabric. So little left of their lives . . . They seem dazed and in some ways hostile . . . Odd, you'd think they'd be glad of the help." Her voice trailed off yet again.

"What's happening now, Lilly?"

"I'm asking Charles about the locals. They don't look too happy to have our help. He's shaking his head . . . abrupt and impatient. 'They've been complaining about our late arrival,' he says.

"'Delays can't be helped on major disasters like this one, but that doesn't make it easier for them — or us,' I tell him.

"'Preaching to the choir, Ms. Santiago. Preaching to the choir.'" Lilly waited for a couple of minutes then continued.

"We're quiet now. Not much to say. Ooh! The trucks are jerking over rough road. We're clinging to the wooden slats. The heavy wet air feels like a weight on my chest. Can't breathe well . . . It's going to be hard on my team. Most of them are from the deserts of Arizona and not used to working in humid conditions."

She turned her head to the side as though trying to focus on some distant sound or vision. Bill waited patiently, letting her continue in her own time.

"We're pulling into the evacuee camp. It's built around a large old building that survived the storm. It's almost bulging from the masses of people crammed inside. . .Her breath came short and shallow. "Oh that's not good . . . not good.

"Hundreds of people are gathered there, squatted down on their heels, suspicious, and watchful. It's going to be tough to gain the trust of these poor people. Some look shell shocked, but others . . . Are we safe here?

"We're stopping now at the housing area. Tent city really is all it is, but I'm used to it.

"'Get your bed assignments and drop your gear. Let's see what we can do to help.'"

When she fell silent and the quiet grew, Bill asked, "Where are you now?"

"It's later. Five . . . five days, I think. We're all dragging into the tents for rest. Everyone's exhausted. I clap my hands. 'Team meeting. Gather around. How's everyone holding up?'

"They are saying okay, but their expressions tell a different tale.

"'Are you having problems with the locals?'

"It's obvious no one wants to complain. 'Linda, what issues are you hitting?'"

"'Well, it's just discouraging. We come all this way to help, but they are really upset that it took so long for us to get here, all I hear is complaints about that.'"

"The others agree. 'That's right,' Hank says. 'When I first get to a new person, they spend the first fifteen minutes telling me we stink because we weren't here when they needed us.'

"'We've been hearing that over and over for days now. People are really upset about how long it is taking to get all the different kinds of help they need,' Susan said.

"'I've been experiencing that myself,' I say. 'How are they once you get past that part?'

"Linda shrugs. 'The ones I talk with seem to appreciate our help. They have all the usual concerns in a situation like this.'

"Hank says they are helping everyone and I agree.

"I smile and try to encourage them but I can feel my stomach flipping. I'm tired and discouraged, too. 'You're all making a difference for these people whether they can see it yet or not. Get some rest and then let's go over to the community center and chat with some of the folks there.'"

Again Lilly rolled her head slowly from side to side as though to see better.

"Where are you now, Lilly? What do you see?"

"Outside the community center. So many people packed into such a tight space. If something happens, they'll never get out.

"There are two children huddled on the sidewalk. I speak to them in Spanish, so I don't frighten them." Lilly twitched slightly like a startled deer ready to flee.

"What is it, Lilly?"

"An explosion or something. Loud . . . cracks . . . like snapping timbers. 'Madré de Dios, run away from here,' I shout at the children and run for the front of the building as they scurry away.

"Masses of people push from the doors, trying desperately to escape. The roof is caving in! The building is collapsing, like slow motion, falling into a pile on top of them.

"I can hear people screaming." A cry came from Lilly, and once again Bill waited. "I see the dust settling and I hear people moaning and sobbing.

"Many hundreds of souls have just lost their lives. Some of my team is in there. I must get them out! We need the search teams STAT. It will take many dozens of people and the dogs to find anyone left alive in the mountain of rubble, I think."

Bill quietly made notes on his tablet as Lilly settled once again into a more peaceful place. "Where are you now, Lilly?"

"It's later . . . a few days . . . a week . . . I don't know. No hope. There's no hope for those inside. The rescue operation is now a recovery mission. A handful of people have been pulled out alive, although seriously injured. The most accurate count is five hundred dead, including three of my people.

"The remaining members of my team are as shell-shocked as the people they came to help, but they won't leave while they're needed. I take a moment's break in the shade of a tree, watching them move among the crowds.

"One of the other volunteer agency team leaders, Barbara Houston, comes over. She looks hot, tired, and agitated.

"'Hi, Barbara. How's it going?'

"'It's not,' she snapped at me. 'I need your team to help us remove the no longer needed sand bags, so we can clean up around here, make it more efficient.'

"'I'm sorry. We're all tied up doing what we can to assist the people with counseling.'

"Barbara's looking at my team and I know she thinks we are just loafing and chatting up the people, not really helping. So much for mental health awareness, I think.

"'Look, I need those bodies cleaning up this mess. I have the power to order done what we need with any volunteers.'

"'I'm sorry, Barbara, but you don't have control over us. We're here to do what we're trained to do. There are immense mental health needs here, especially with the building collapse. I'm really sorry, but we can't help you right now.'

"'I'm going to go find the Director. You'll be sorry about this. You're no team player and that's what we need down here. We don't have time for prima donnas!'

"She's stomping off, headed in the direction of the Director's communication tent. The disaster is taking a toll on everyone."

"All right, Lilly. You're doing fine. Take another deep breath and relax a bit deeper. You're safe here . . .Where are you now?"

"Hank is coming. 'We need to talk. Can we go over there away from these people?'

"'What's up?'

"'I don't know how to say this.'

"'What?'

"'I was just talking with Barbara and Jim. He was trying to cool her down, but I felt I had to tell you what I heard.'

"'If she's trying to get me into hot water, it won't be the first time.'

"Hank's jaw's tight and he's frowning. This must be serious. 'It's worse than that. She was ranting and raving. Really carrying on.' He's hesitating, afraid to speak up. 'Go on, Hank.' 'She told him that she planned to kill you.'

"'That can't be right. Why would she say such a thing?'

"'I don't know, but she said she's going to stab you with rebar from the building collapse and then slit your throat with her knife. She said "that bitch won't know what hit her."'

"'Oh my, that does put a pretty serious spin on it, doesn't it?'

"'What are we going to do?'

"'Right now, you and I are going somewhere to sit down and talk about this. Then I will worry about her.'"

Lilly plucked at the quilt with her fingertips, then her hands stilled in her lap. "I'm back in my tent. I can't stop shaking. What am I going to do? I know Barbara has access to the salvage material and all of us carry knives for emergencies. Was she unstable enough to carry out her threat? I'm disgusted with the site supervisor. He is no help at all. I am so afraid."

Lilly started to shake again. "Lilly, everything is ok, I am going to count from ten to one and you will slowly be back in my office, safe, warm, and relaxed," Bill said. "Coming all the way back, now." He snapped his fingers when he reached one.

Her eyes flicked open, and she sat clenching and unclenching her fists. "My hands are numb."

"That's okay. You were under quite a while and that happens. Would you like some water?"

"Yes, please." She sat up and looked at Bill expectantly.

He knew from reports supplied by Lilly's team that they were concerned about her and had been concerned about Barbara's threat. It was her team that demanded she be flown on a medevac flight to the hospital where she now was.

"Lilly, I'd say you have good reason to be afraid and stressed. We'll work through this together."

Ethical Points to Consider:

Lilly is experiencing a number of issues. First and foremost, returning to a psychologically healthy state. In terms of ethics, there is a duty to warn issue (ACA, 2005; APA, 2002; NAADAC, 2008; & NASW, 2008). In this instance, the mental health supervisor is the intended victim. The counselor appropriately warned her regarding the threat. Although Barbara has made a threat, has access to a weapon, and opportunity, it does not appear the managers of the relief efforts pulled her off assignment to ensure the safety of Lilly. Lilly is left to decide whether to stay on the job and keep herself safe, or leave. The counselor who warned Lilly should confront the managers with the concern regarding Lilly's safety. Contacting the police may become necessary if the situation continues to be downplayed. As it turns out, Lilly leaves on mental health emergency basis.

In this case, we are reminded of the need for mental health professionals to engage in self-care. Lilly appears stressed out almost before the job begins. Once her life is threatened, her stress levels escalate tenfold. Ethical codes increasingly are calling upon mental health professionals to engage in self-care and mandating they not practice when impaired due to stress, psychological disorder, etc. (ACA, 2005; APA, 2002; NAADAC, 2008; & NASW, 2008). Prior to returning to work, Lilly must heal herself. It will be critical she learn coping strategies to help her during future disasters. The organization also needs to develop strategies to address workers who threaten others.

Discussion Questions:

1. What are Lilly's cognitions, emotions, and behaviors? Given your identification of these issues, what theoretical orientation will guide your work with her?

2. Explain whether short- or long-term therapy would be most beneficial for Lilly. Outline how treatment should proceed.

3. Does Lilly qualify for a diagnosis? If so, with what disorder(s)? What is her global assessment of functioning scores for: pre-disaster, admission, and her appointment with Bill?

4. How might diagnosing Lilly impact her volunteer work, mental health license, and ability to obtain malpractice insurance?

5. As a consultant, how would you convince the volunteer agency to place their volunteer's safety and health as a high priority?

6. How would you recommend preventing burnout and vicarious trauma among mental health professionals doing disaster work? Develop a personal plan to mitigate these processes in yourself.

7. What duty to warn and involuntary commitment issues were at work here? What, if anything, would you have changed in the response made to the threat?

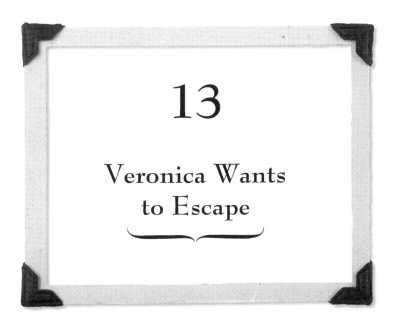

13

Veronica Wants to Escape

For Your Consideration

As you read about Veronica and her experiences, be aware of your biases with respect to the case and how they impact your interpretation of the case. Consider whether a diagnosis is appropriate. Various treatment options exist and could be provided from different theoretical orientations. Consider which would be best and why. Finally, what cultural and ethical issues are critical to address?

Veronica's Story

Veronica woke with a start, sweat dripping down her face. Her heart raced and her breaths came fast and shallow. She glanced at her husband, Greg, afraid she had awakened him, but he slept soundly beside her. Tossing back the blankets, she rose and went to the bathroom for a glass of water.

She hated this dream, hated her fear. Would these nightmares never stop? When Veronica thought of her silly apprehensions, she couldn't help but think of the courage her parents had shown in fleeing Vietnam in small, barely sea worthy boats. They had persevered and made it to the shores of the United States thirty-five years earlier. Veronica was the first of the family to be born in America.

Veronica downed the last of the water and stared at her reflection in the mirror. She knew her classic Asian looks had landed her a place as one of the top models in the country and brought international jobs as well. Lately though, her fears were increasing, and she turned down more jobs than she accepted.

She jumped and spun around when Greg's face appeared in the mirror next to hers. Her heart jumped into overdrive yet again.

"Hey, Babe, you have another dream?" He ran his hands up and down her arms, warming her chilled skin. When she simply nodded, he coaxed her back to bed to warm herself under the covers.

"What was it this time, Roni?" he asked, using his pet name for her.

"Same thing. Worse this time. I couldn't move. I was so humiliated." She shuddered against his body. "I don't want to think about it anymore. Let's talk about something else."

He pulled her tight against the curve of his body, hugging her close to warm her. "How about kids? Want to talk about the possibility of starting a family?"

She frowned into the dark room. Was she ready? Could she offer a good mother to the children they brought into the world?

"I don't know, Greg. Do you think we're ready?"

"Well, you're staying home more, not taking on so many jobs. Maybe it is a natural progression to wanting to be a stay-at-home mom."

"Could be," she said quietly. "Let's think about it a while longer. I think a baby might be just the thing for us, though." Her frown turned into a gentle smile. "It would be lovely to create a little being between the two of us, wouldn't it?"

"I love you," Greg said. "I want to start a family with you."

She sighed and let him pull her into an embrace.

The next morning, Veronica made her way to the local market with a long list of necessities. It had been so long since she'd gone shopping, the cupboards were bare and the freezer drained of any possibilities. When she grasped the cart and walked through the sliding doors, her palms instantly started to sweat. Her breath hitched in her chest. "You are all right," she mumbled. "Get a grip and get it done fast. You are just fine."

She hurried up and down the first three rows. In the fourth, several women clustered, their carts clogging the way. When she turned to go around the other direction, two more had come behind her.

"Excuse me." Nothing, they continued looking at the shelves. "Excuse me," she said more loudly. "I have to get by. Please." Her tone pleaded and finally one of the women moved her cart aside in time to see Veronica abandon her half-filled cart and race past.

At her Jaguar, she dropped into the low slung car, leaning her forehead against the steering wheel and gasping for air.

With tears streaming down her face, she turned the key, started the engine and pointed the car toward home.

"What do you mean you didn't get any food?" Greg's voice raised, and she knew he was fighting his frustration. "I've gotten food the last three times. What's the matter with you?"

"I don't know, Greg. I get inside the store, and I can't stay. I simply can't stay in there. I have to come home. I'm not sure it would matter to me if I never leave this house again."

"Where have you been during the days you haven't worked lately?" Now he sounded puzzled.

She shrugged. "I haven't been anywhere. I've stayed home mostly."

"Doing what? You always loved to be going out, staying busy."

"Oh, this and that. Cleaning house. Reading. Staying up on the industry."

"What's the point of that," he burst out. "You haven't accepted a job in six months." With a heavy sigh he dropped his chin to his chest. "What's wrong, Veronica? I want to help you."

"I don't know, Greg. I wish I did. I feel safe here, loved. Out there," she nodded toward their front picture window, "I'm afraid, like someone is after me . . . I just can't run fast enough . . . or something . . . I don't know. I just don't know." She turned and ran sobbing from the room.

Two days later, Greg buttoned his shirt after having his blood pressure checked. "Hey, doc, can I ask you something about my wife?" he asked his long time physician.

"Sure. What's the problem?"

"I'm not sure. I think she needs a shrink or something. You know she's an international runway model?"

The doctor nodded. "I've seen her pictures. She's a beautiful woman. So what's the problem?"

"Lately she isn't taking really good job offers and doesn't want to leave the house. She's having nightmares, too."

"Sounds like it's out of my realm, unless you think something is going on physically?"

"I don't think so. She seems healthy enough, other than her fears."

Doctor Wilkerson grabbed a prescription pad and scribbled out a name and phone number. "This is a colleague of mine. Excellent therapist. Why don't you ask her to call him?"

Greg took the slip of paper and read the name Stanley Shapiro. Maybe this is just what she needs, he thought. "Thanks, Doc. We'll do it."

It was a week before Stanley could see Veronica. Greg went with her the first time to be sure she got there. On the ride to the office, Veronica fidgeted in her seat, tugging at the hem of her skirt and wishing she could get Greg to turn around and take her home. She'd tried making the excuse of feeling ill. He wasn't buying it.

Greg pulled into a parking space. "Do you want me to go in or just wait here?"

She thought for a minute, wondering if there was any chance she could get out of this. "No, you can wait here if you want. I'll be fine." She leaned into him for a quick kiss and then climbed out of the car.

After twenty minutes, she made it up the elevator. On the third floor of the medical building she found Dr. Shapiro's office and stepped into the waiting room. A secretary asked her to have a seat and fill out what seemed like reams of paper. She had barely handed it back to the grey haired woman when the inner door opened and a handsome blonde walked out and invited her inside. When she passed him, he shook her hand and greeted her with a warm and welcoming smile.

"Dr. Shapiro, I don't know if I really need to be here. I'm really happy."

"Come on in and have a seat. Let's just chat, all right?"

She shrugged. She was already here, why not play along with Greg. Maybe it would make him happy.

"All right, thanks." She glanced around the room and took an isolated chair, choosing to avoid the clichéd couch. Dr. Shapiro sat opposite her.

"Dr. Shapiro —"

"Call me Stanley if you like, Mrs. Branford."

"Okay, and I'm just Veronica."

"I don't believe anyone is just anything. Tell me how I can help you." His smile seemed genuine, and she began to relax a bit.

"My husband thinks I have a problem."

"Do you think you do?"

"Maybe, I don't know."

"What's been going on for you?"

A vision flashed through her head, the nightmare again, and her breath hitched in her throat. "It all started when I stopped accepting modeling jobs."

"Don't you like modeling?"

Her face lit up. She didn't have to see it to know that it had. She loved the runway. She also knew she was good at what she did.

"It's not that. I love it. The travel, the glamour, the clothes."

"So why have you stopped doing something you obviously love?"

"I'm afraid," she barely whispered it.

"I'm sorry. Did you say you're afraid?"

She nodded and looked down where her hands were folded in her lap.

"What is it that frightens you?"

"I keep having these thoughts. I'm falling on the runway, and I can't stop the fall. Everyone is just staring at me and I can't move. It's as though I'm frozen there."

"Have you ever tripped on the runway?"

"Oh sure. We all do sooner or later, but I've never fallen."

"You hesitate. What else is bothering you?"

"It all started with the dream, doing fewer jobs, now...."

"Now?"

"I don't want to leave my apartment. I'm safe there. I'm afraid to go outside."

"Are you afraid someone will harm you there?"

"Yes, I suppose so. I go into stores or businesses and if too many people are there, I just freak out and have to go home. I can't stay. So I get home as fast as I can and close myself in."

"Is anyone making you feel like you want to hide? How about your husband?"

She smiled then, but it faded to a frown. "I love my husband, but things are getting pretty strained. He is frustrated, and he's had to take over all the chores like shopping and picking up dry cleaning since I rarely go out."

"Is there anyone else you fear from inside the family?"

Veronica thought of her mother, of the demands that she and Greg start a family and provide grandchildren. "When I'm in, I don't answer the phone or the door. I ignore them and let Greg handle anything important when he comes home."

"Why? Who do you not want to talk to?"

"My mother."

"Have you two had a falling out?"

"Not really." Veronica sighed. "She is pushing me to start a family with Greg, and I want to get this issue of being housebound taken care of first. How can I take proper care of a child when I can't even take a baby outside or to the doctor? I can't take care of myself at this point let alone a helpless child." She sighed. "I feel helpless to fight this."

"Veronica, we'll gradually work at getting you back out into the world a little at a time. You will come to see that it is okay to be a little anxious and that nothing will happen to you. We'll also work on setting some boundaries on choices that are rightfully yours and your husband's. How does that sound?"

Her stomach tightened at the thought of going out. "I don't know. I think I'm afraid."

"We can do this together and I can teach your husband how to help you, too, when you both want to go to a movie or dinner. What do you say?"

Veronica clamped her lips together. She was tired of giving away her control and power. "All right. How do we start?"

Stanley picked up an appointment book. "Can you be here tomorrow at three?"

She gave a sardonic laugh. "I don't have anything else to do."

"Will you be able to come to the office again?"

"I think so."

"Just remember, you will be all right. Do some self-talk to reassure yourself and stay determined to be here. Know that there is an answer to this, and I'll do all I can to get you through it. But you have to work hard, too."

"All right. I'll try." Veronica rose and shook hands with Stanley. A frisson of electricity danced up her arm, and she found herself drawn to the bluest eyes she had ever seen. She pulled her hand out of his and left the office without a backward glance.

Veronica attended her first two appointments, but when the outings and assignments from Stanley became tougher, she missed several in a row. She had just finished cancelling a fifth appointment with his secretary when the phone rang. She reached for it, but then stopped, waiting for the machine to take it.

"Veronica? This is Stanley. Are you listening? I want you to answer the phone for me."

With a sigh she picked up the receiver. "I'm here," she said quietly.

"I understand you just cancelled on me again. You were my last one of the day. How about I come to you, and we go out for a walk?"

"I don't know." Other than seeing Stanley, she hadn't been out at all since those first few appointments.

"Veronica?"

"All right. Do you know where we live?"

"I do. Be there in thirty minutes. Don't change your mind on me now. Why don't you sit down, do some deep breathing and listen to the mediation music I gave you until I get there?"

"All right." She carefully replaced the receiver and wished she were anywhere but there, for more reasons than one.

When she opened the front door to Stanley a short time later, the sunlight bounced off blond highlights in his hair. It accentuated the blue of his eyes, and she felt a pull toward him. She forced that aside, knowing she was just feeling lonely since Greg had become distant during the past few months.

"Come in, Stanley."

They went into the living room and talked for a few minutes. Veronica told him she'd been unable to go even to the post office since their last meeting.

"Let's go to the little park I saw right on the corner," he suggested.

She shook her head automatically, but when his face lit up with a reassuring smile, she gave in.

Together they walked down the sidewalk toward the lush green grass and plentiful wild flowers of the local park. When an elderly couple came toward them, she started to turn back, but Stanley caught her elbow and whispered reassuringly to her until they had passed by. At the park a lone man sat reading a book under a shade tree. When Stanley tried to lead her along the path toward the man, she blatantly refused to go there and swung around toward home. They'd been gone only ten minutes but she had to get back to safety. She could feel it.

Over the weeks that followed, Stanley and Veronica made many more forays into the neighborhood, finally into the community at large. He made her feel safe, and he was patient, not as demanding as Greg had become. Stanley seemed to her to be a knight in shining armor ready to protect and defend.

On one particularly long trip out, Veronica admitted to herself she was falling for Stanley. She knew she loved Greg, so how could that be? She was getting better about going out, although it still helped to have either Stanley or Greg with her. As she looked at Stanley and questioned where their relationship could go, she could see he was only interested in her professionally, and she did love Greg. It was time to end the counseling relationship and continue working on her problems alone.

Ethical Points to Consider:

In this case, we find a client who is attracted to her therapist and wondering how far their relationship can go. For the sake of argument, we will assume Stanley, the counselor, is aware of the attraction and it is mutual, although not to the extent Veronica feels. Ethical codes are clear in prohibiting sexual relationships with clients (ACA, 2005; APA, 2002; NAADAC, 2008; & NASW, 2008). The codes are also clear that clients are not to be exploited or used to meet the mental health worker's needs (ACA, 2005; APA, 2002; NAADAC, 2008; & NASW, 2008). Moreover, dual relationships must be avoided (ACA, 2005; APA, 2002; NAADAC, 2008; & NASW, 2008).

The counselor has some decisions to make. This is a situation in which to seek supervision. If the attraction is only the client's and not strong, the therapist may be able to work through it in session. If it is a strong attraction by the client, the therapist may need to refer. Attraction to a client by his/her therapist needs to be explored by the therapist, preferably in supervision or consultation. What is triggering/causing the attraction? How strong is it? Can the therapist effectively work with the client? If necessary, how will the therapist terminate and refer? Supervision and self-reflection help to determine whether the attraction is tied to someone the client reminds the counselor of, how strong the attraction is, and whether the attraction can be set aside to allow counseling to continue. In other instances, the attraction may be very strong and the client should be referred.

Discussion Questions:

1. What are Veronica's key cognitions, emotions, and behaviors that you will integrate into your counseling? Given your identification of these issues, what theoretical orientation would you choose in your work with her? How do you conceptualize the case? What specific techniques and treatment plan would you employ?

2. How might her cultural background and societal expectations affect Veronica? How will they affect your work with her?

3. What, if any, diagnosis would you make? What symptoms support your diagnosis?

4. Would you recommend couples counseling? Why or why not?

5. How might Veronica's work as a model impact her current choices and situation?

6. How would you handle Veronica's attraction to Stanley? What would you do if the attraction was mutual, but not acted upon?

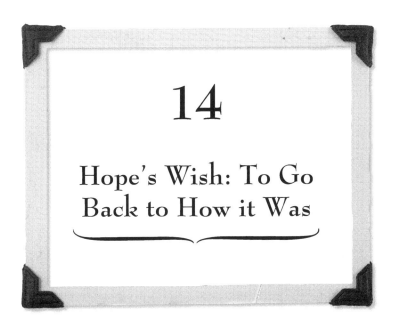

14

Hope's Wish: To Go Back to How it Was

For Your Consideration

As you read about Hope and her experiences, be aware of your reactions and biases with respect to her situation and how they impact your interpretation of the case. Consider what you would recommend for each member of her family. Multiple treatment options exist and could be provided from a variety of professional fields. Consider what you would recommend for treatment and why? Finally, how does your experience and knowledge of family therapy impact your recommendations?

Hope's Story

Hope swerved into the center lane, away from the bicycling man. Her heart raced and her breath gasped.

"Did I hit him? Look out back. Is he in the road?"

Two of her children looked at each other and exchanged a look she caught in the rear view mirror. She ignored it and shrieked again, "Are the twins ok? Did I hit him?"

"Yes, Mom, they are still safely buckled in their car seats," her son Anthony replied. "You didn't hit the guy on the bike, didn't even get close."

Hope heard the disgusted tone in the eleven-year-old's voice and knew he was tired of her questions, her suspicions — but she couldn't help it.

She made a hard right turn around the corner, racing down the road and making another right, and then right again. She had to go back, had to see for herself whether she hit the cyclist or not.

"Mom, how come you never trust us?" her six-year-old asked. "We wouldn't lie to you."

Sandy sounded pouty, but at the same time the question seemed to come from a child much older than her chronological years. Hope knew her children were growing up in anything but a normal home, and two years ago when the twins arrived, it got even crazier.

Hope's hands shook and her heart continued to race as she slowly drove past the place she believed she had hit the man. He was nowhere to be seen. As relief flowed through her, a tear slipped from the corner of her eye to be quickly followed by a flood of them. Why did she believe such things?

"We told you, you missed him, Mom. Can we go to the store now?" Anthony asked.

She simply nodded yes and drove slowly down the main road of their small town. Every car that passed them, every person standing on the street corners drew her attention. Did she know them? Were they from here or the nearby town with its population of drug users?

Hope forced the thoughts away as well as she could. She deliberately lightened her tone. "What do you say to some ice cream and cookies for desert tonight?"

Both children chimed in with their approval and after parking, they got out of the sparkling clean car and hurried toward the store. Hope watched them and knew they wanted in and out of the place as much as she did.

Together they moved down the aisles, her son pushing the cart down the exact center of the aisle, and her daughter taking the things off the shelves and placing them in the basket at her direction. Hope kept her hands carefully folded across the large expanse of her belly.

As Sandy reached for a box of macaroni and cheese, Hope snapped, "No! Not that one."

The girl's shoulders drooped, and she sighed. "Which one, Mommy?"

"I'm sorry, sweetie. Get the second from the left. That's a good one."

"'Kay."

Hope saw the glance between her two children. She ignored it as much as she could. She knew she was making their lives a living hell, but couldn't stop herself.

"Come on, let's get those cookies and ice cream, and we'll get out of here and go home," she said.

At the ice cream freezer, she stopped and stared. "Anthony, is that Mrs. Tolliver from Centerville?"

He dutifully gazed at the older woman and then shook his head. "No. I don't know her."

"Are you sure?"

"I'm sure."

"Go ask her name."

"Aw, Mom . . ."

Hope gave him a nudge. "Go on. Please. For me."

She watched him approach the grey-haired lady and moved so she could see whether or not Anthony touched the woman or her cart.

He walked back to her shaking his head. "She's not from here. She's a snow bird from Wisconsin and just got into town."

"Are you sure she's telling the truth?"

"Yes, she is. She thought we were being neighborly by asking about her." He shook his head as though wondering at the minds of old people and how they thought.

The woman reached into the freezer and pulled a carton of their favorite ice cream out. Hope groaned.

"I don't like the ice cream here," she said to Anthony and Sandra after a brief hesitation. "Let's go get some from the ice cream shop. We'll splurge just this once."

Sandy clapped her hands together and bounced. "Oh, boy, we never get to go there."

Hope smiled at her little one. "Today we will. It will be a special treat."

"Right," Anthony muttered.

A short time later, they pulled into the strip mall and parked away from the entrance to the shop. Hope slid her gaze over all the cars, over couples sitting at tables outside. Thank God, no one I know, she thought.

"Anthony take the cash and get whatever you two want and something for the twins. I'd like a waffle cone with vanilla and blueberries."

"Right, Mommy," said Sandy. "We'll get it."

"Take her hand," she called out to her son as they started across the pavement.

She watched him glance at the parking lot, not a moving car in sight and shake his head. The kids didn't know what to make of her, she knew, even after growing up with her and her eccentricities.

A happy couple smiled at each other like newlyweds. Hope tried to remember what it was like to be loved so much. To be forgiven anything, even illness. She shook her head. She couldn't even think back to what it was like when she and Jonathan had first married. Her problems had been manageable then. They hadn't escalated until she had gotten pregnant with Anthony. His birth seemed to be the spark that started her down this path of destruction.

Hope sighed at the memory of his first word, his first shaky step. She and Jonathan had delighted in all of his accomplishments, and her illness seemed to subside. And then she got pregnant again. After the second child, the symptoms worsened and she lost control.

Loneliness overwhelmed her, and once again tears gathered in her eyes. There's no hope for me, she thought. No one can help me. Without Medicare disability to pay for my meds, I'd be on the street or in a psych ward someplace. She knew the kids hated begging at the Salvation Army for vouchers to pay for utilities and using the food stamp card was a huge embarrassment for them, but it was the best she could do since Jonathan gave up and left them.

She forced her thoughts aside and smiled at the kids when they came back carrying their cones.

"Thanks, Mom," Anthony said as he climbed in. "This is great."

"Yummy," Sandy agreed around licks.

Hope laughed for the first time that day. "You're welcome. Chow down and then we'll go home and get this food put up."

Anthony and Sandy seemed to savor every bite, or procrastinate in light of the coming chores, Hope wasn't sure which. It didn't matter. It was the first relaxed moment they had had in a week. She would let them enjoy it while it lasted.

Hope pulled into the drive, stopped, then backed up two feet. She looked around her yard and driveway as the kids waited for her signal to jump out. A paper blew from the back of the yard near the garbage cans, across the driveway, and Hope put the car in reverse and swung it around to another part of the drive, stopping again and watching to see which way the paper traveled.

"This is good," she said at last. "Let's unload."

She saw Anthony send Sandy a "that-means-we'll-unload" look. "Sorry, kids. Let's get it done and then you can play or watch a movie."

The kids grabbed bags, and Hope led the way through the front yard, weaving around bushes and rocks, avoiding areas that weren't safe for them to step on.

At the door, she used her house key to turn the lock and the handle, opening the door without touching it. "Kick your shoes off," she said as her own sandals hit the dirt and stayed outside, allowing her to enter barefoot.

Like a sentinel, she stood and watched Anthony and Sandy bringing in bag after bag until the car was empty and the kitchen counters were full. They worked together to get everything put away in the limited space they had.

"Mom, when are we going to clean those two cabinets out so we can use them?" Anthony asked.

She looked at the closed doors, enemies to be sure, knowing legal papers from the courthouse lay behind them. A fine sweat broke out on her forehead and her heart rate picked up. "Soon, Anthony, soon I hope."

With a heavy sigh, he shook his head and walked away to his room. Sandy was off and running for her bedroom and games. At least they could get away from her there, in their private spaces. They would take the twins, as always, and watch them for their mom.

Despair flowed over her at the thought that her children had to hide from her to get any peace in their own home. Maybe I should just kill myself and let Jonathan take them. I'm no good to them like this. She shook off the thought as well as she could and picked up a soda.

Moving into the tiny living room, Hope sat in her easy chair, the cold drink in her hand. She absently ran her fingertips over the scar on her head. The remnants of the accident that nearly killed her created a dull ache from time to time in her shoulder, and today was no exception.

Her gaze fell on the note card lying on the end table at her side. It was from her aunt in Hilo, Hawaii. Anthony had opened and read it to her, a decision she regretted as soon as he read the content. Her aunt was writing to let her know that her offer to move there was still open. Aunt Elizabeth really believed that being in a new location for awhile would give Hope the respite she needed. Hope wondered at the demons that drove her crazy. Was it possible to be somewhere where they didn't run her life?

What a messed up life, she thought, clicking on the television. Time to lose herself in some senseless show, time to try to pass one more day without further fear — if she could.

At six that evening, Jonathan stopped by to drop off money for the bills. When he stepped into the living room, his gaze slid around the edges. The furniture in the center was spotless, newly oiled wood. The corner pieces were a different story. There's enough dust on those to grow tomatoes, he thought, shaking his head in disgust. How can she live like this? How had he ever lived like this? he wondered.

"Have a seat, Jonathan. The kids will be out in a minute."

He glanced around again wondering where it was safe to sit. "Where?" he snapped.

"The loveseat's fine."

He slumped onto it and set a new envelope of cash on the coffee table. "This has to last for two weeks. I missed a few days of work."

"Thanks, it'll help. What was wrong? Are you better now?"

"Just a flu bug," he said, and nodded as she called for Anthony and Sandy to come and see their dad.

"Anthony, grab your dad a soda, would you?" she asked when the two came down the hall.

"Sure." He went into the kitchen and brought a bottle back with him as Sandy jumped into her dad's lap.

"Here you go, Dad."

Anthony handed him the bottle and went to stand beside his mother, protective, a bit defensive, Jonathan wasn't sure.

"Hey son, can you give us a minute?"

Anger seemed to radiate from the boy. "You have a problem?" Jonathan asked him. Sandy slid off his lap and moved away, seeming to sense trouble coming.

Anthony opened his mouth as though to speak, but shut it again. "No, no I don't." He turned on his heel and stalked to his room, slamming the door behind him. Sandy ran down the hall after him and let herself into his room without knocking.

"What's up with that?" Jonathan asked Hope.

She shrugged. "He misses you and I think he resents that you left him to deal with me and my — issues."

Jonathan looked at the cold bottle in his hand, fought the retort that wanted to jump from his throat. "What's going on, Hope?"

"I've thought about going to Hilo for awhile, it might help. If things are better there, the kids could join me in a few months."

"Just moving isn't going to make your — issues — go away, is it?"

"No, probably not. But my aunt has a counselor who can try some different meds and therapies. He's actually had some success with people like me. I need to go it alone for the first few months."

He watched the color drain from her face as she thought about it, but knew she wanted a normal life for all of them. He couldn't watch her slide down her personal path to hell anymore. Especially since he and the kids had to go with her.

Slowly he stood and set his now empty bottle down. "I think it's a good idea, but I know it would be a really tough choice for you. Anyway, I have to go now. We'll talk more soon."

Fear shimmied across her features. "When will you come see them? Will you move there, too?"

He chewed his lip. "I don't know, Hope. I don't know if I can. My job is here. Say goodbye to the kids for me."

Jonathan turned abruptly and walked out, leaving the front door standing open in his wake. He knew she wouldn't want him to touch the outside of it. Someone would close it from inside when it got too cold to leave it open.

Six Months Later

The phone rang and Anthony and Sandy raced to grab it first. It was the day and time their mom always called. When Anthony beat her to the living room phone, Sandy scurried into the kitchen and grabbed that one.

"Hi, Mom," they shouted with joy.

"Hey kids, I miss you so much. I love it here in Paradise and know someday you will be here with me. You'll love it, too. You can swim and play in the ocean, all kinds of things."

"Mom, you wouldn't believe how well we are doing in school, but we miss you all the time. That makes it hard," Anthony said.

"I miss you, too, but the medication and counseling are helping. We will see each other soon and maybe we can live like a normal family." Hope sighed. "Anyway, are you watching out for the twins?"

"Yeah, they're doin' great," Sandy said. "Dad is helping us with our work, too."

Sometime Later

The Boeing jet touched down at Hilo. Hope peered eagerly out the large glass windows, straining to see what she could from her place behind the security barrier. After what seemed like hours, Hope saw

Sandy, Anthony and the twins come past the guards and she wrapped them in a group hug.

Anthony looked unsure of her and seemed afraid something would spoil the moment.

"Just like I told you on the phone, honey, the medication and counseling have really helped. I feel so much better than before."

Anthony and Sandy grinned from ear to ear. Maybe life would be great for the reunited family — in Paradise — for at least awhile.

Ethical Points to Consider:

When children are involved, the mental health worker evaluates that they are not being neglected or abused. In this case, the mental health worker might be asked to provide a recommendation regarding the ability of the mother to care for her children. Are the children neglected or in danger? Here we find parents who live at great distances from one another. If custody were to become an issue, the counselor must remember that courts decide custody and it is a legal matter. Often, however, mental health workers are asked to provide an opinion regarding parenting skills. It is important that the statements focus only on what the counselor has evaluated and observed. Moreover, only statements regarding the parent the counselor worked with should be made. That is, if the counselor has not had contact with one of the parents, his/her only knowledge of the parent is via statements made by the children or spouse. Any of this information must be properly documented as to the source.

Discussion Questions:

1. What are Hope's cognitions, emotions, and behaviors? Which of her actions do you consider abnormal or outside of the typical range? Given your viewpoints, what theoretical orientation will guide your work with her? What diversity factors impact your case conceptualization?

2. Do Hope or others in her family meet any diagnostic criteria for a mental disorder? If so, what disorder(s)?

3. How might you incorporate her estranged husband in treatment?

4. What are Hope's options?

5. What, if any, is the impact of the car accident?

6. How might trust issues be involved with treatment?

7. What are your recommendations regarding her children? What ethical concerns do you have regarding her ability to parent? Where do you believe the children should reside? If they were to continue to reside with the father, do you see a decline in Hope's symptoms?

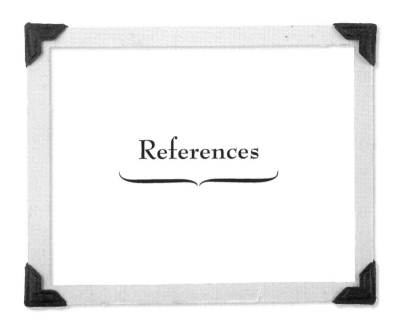

References

American Counseling Association (ACA). (2005). *ACA code of ethics.* Alexandria, VA: Author.

American Psychological Association (APA). (2002). *Ethical principles of psychologists and code of conduct.* Washington, DC: Author.

Bennett, B. E., Bricklin, P. M., Harris, E., Knapp, S., VandeCreek, L., & Younggren, J. N. (2006). *Assessing and managing risk in psychological practice: An individualized approach.* Rockville, MD: The Trust.

National Association for Alcoholism and Drug Abuse Counselors (NAADAC). (2008). *NAADAC code of ethics.* Alexandria, VA: Author.

National Association of Social Workers (NASW). (2008). *Code of ethics of the national association of social workers.* Washington, DC: Author.

Remley, T. P., & Herlihy, B. (2007). *Ethical, legal and professional issues in counseling* (2nd ed.). Upper Saddle River, NJ: Pearson.

```
STUDY PACKAGE
CONTINUING EDUCATION
CREDIT INFORMATION
```

CASE STUDIES IN ETHICS, DIAGNOSIS & TREATMENT

Thank you for choosing PESI, LLC as your continuing education provider. Our goal is to provide you with current, accurate and practical information from the most experienced and knowledgeable speakers and authors.

Listed below are the continuing education credit(s) currently available for this self-study package. *Please note: Your state licensing board dictates whether self study is an acceptable form of continuing education. Please refer to your state rules and regulations.*

COUNSELORS: CMI Education Institute, Inc. is recognized by the National Board for Certified Counselors to offer continuing education for National Certified Counselors. Provider #: 5637. We adhere to NBCC Continuing Education Guidelines. This self-study package qualifies for **3.0** contact hours.

SOCIAL WORKERS: CMI Education Institute, Inc., 1062, is approved as a provider for social work continuing education by the Association of Social Work Boards (ASWB), 400 South Ridge Parkway, Suite B, Culpeper VA 22701. www.aswb.org. CMI Education Institute, Inc. maintains responsibility for the program. Licensed Social Workers should contact their regulatory board to determine course approval. Social Workers will receive **3.0** (Ethical) continuing education clock hours for completing this self-study package. Course Level: All Levels.

PSYCHOLOGISTS: CMI Education Institute, Inc. is approved by the American Psychological Association to sponsor continuing education for psychologists. CMI Education Institute, Inc. maintains responsibility for these materials and their content. CMI Education Institute, Inc. is offering these self-study materials for **3.0** hours of continuing education credit.

MARRIAGE & FAMILY THERAPISTS: This activity consists of **3.0** clock hours of continuing education instruction. Credit requirements and approvals vary per state board regulations. Please save the course outline, the certificate of completion you receive from the activity and contact your state board or organization to determine specific filing requirements.

ADDICTION COUNSELORS: CMI Education Institute, Inc. is a Provider approved by NAADAC Approved Education Provider Program. Provider #: 00131. This self-study package qualifies for **3.5** contact hours.

Procedures:
1. Review the material.
2. If seeking credit, complete the posttest/evaluation form:

   - Complete posttest/evaluation in entirety, including your email address to receive your certificate much faster versus by mail.

   - Upon completion, mail to the address listed on the form along with the CE fee stated on the test. Tests will not be processed without the CE fee included.

   - Completed posttests must be received 6 months from the date of purchase.

Your completed posttest/evaluation will be graded. If you receive a passing score (70% and above), you will be emailed/faxed/mailed a certificate of successful completion with earned continuing education credits. (Please write your email address on the posttest/evaluation form for fastest response.) If you do not pass the posttest, you will be sent a letter indicating areas of deficiency, and another posttest to complete. The posttest must be resubmitted and receive a passing grade before credit can be awarded. We will allow you to re-take as many times as necessary to receive a certificate.
If you have any questions, please feel free to contact our customer service department at 1.800.844.8260.

CMI Education Institute, Inc.

A Non-Profit Organization Connecting Knowledge with Need Since 1979

  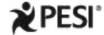

CMI Education
PO BOX 1000
Eau Claire, WI 54702-1000

CASE STUDIES IN ETHICS, DIAGNOSIS & TREATMENT

 CMI Education Institute, Inc.
A Non-Profit Organization Connecting Knowledge with Need Since 1979

  PESI

Any persons interested in receiving credit may photocopy this form, complete and return with a payment of $15.00 per person CE fee. A certificate of successful completion will be sent to you. To receive your certificate sooner than two weeks, rush processing is available for a fee of $10. Please attach check or include credit card information below.

Mail to: PESI, PO Box 1000, Eau Claire, WI 54702

CE Fee: $15: (Rush processing fee: $10)

Total to be charged _____

Credit Card #: _____

Exp Date: _____ **V-Code*:** _____
(*MC/VISA/Discover: last 3-digit # on signature panel on back of card.)
(*American Express: 4-digit # above account # on face of card.)

Name (please print): _____

Address: _____ City: _____

State: _____ Zip Code: _____

Daytime Phone: _____

Signature: _____

Email: _____

Date Completed: _____

Actual time (# of hours) taken to complete this offering: _____ hours

Program Objectives
After completing this publication, I have been able to achieve these objectives:

Identify the critical client and therapy issues.	Yes	No
Apply ethical codes to real-life situation.	Yes	No
Explain accurate reporting of test results.	Yes	No
Recognize confidentiality violations and how to avoid them.	Yes	No

CMI Education
PO BOX 1000
Eau Claire, WI 54702-1000

ZNT041320

CE Release Date: 4/19/10

800-554-9775

Participant Profile:
1. Job Title: _____ Employment setting: _____

1. Reporting child abuse in the distant past is mandated by all states.
a. TRUE
b. FALSE

2. In regard to informed consent when providing counseling to minors:
a. Only the parents are provided with it
b. Only the child is provided with it
c. At least one parent/guardian, if not both, and the child are provided with informed consent
d. None of the above

3. Violation of confidentiality exists when reporting test data and diagnoses to faculty at a   university so that they may provide appropriate accommodation.
a. TRUE
b. FALSE

4. No violation of confidentiality ever occurs when approaching a client with their spouse in a public setting to say hello.
a. TRUE
b. FALSE

5. Informed consent:
a. Must be in age-appropriate language the child understands
b. Must be provided to the parent/guardian(s)
c. Must be provided to the child and parent/guardian(s) in age-appropriate language that all clearly understand

6. Rights to educational records:
a. Vary and may extend to the parents beyond the son/daughter's age of 18
b. Are clear in prohibiting universities from releasing any records to parents
c. Include mental health case notes when filed in a different location from the student's academic record

7. No states mandate reporting impaired drivers
a. TRUE
b. FALSE

8. Accurate reporting of test results:
a. Includes raw and scaled scores, and interpretation
b. Includes test questions, scores, and interpretation
c. Includes individual question answers, test questions and interpretation

9. When providing information about a client (for example, to the courts), it is important to focus on the client as well as interpretations of his/her family members who are not clients
a. TRUE
b. FALSE

10. It is acceptable to ask clients for discounts on items they sell (for example, a discount on a car or reduced sales commission
a. TRUE
b. FALSE

CMI Education
PO BOX 1000
Eau Claire, WI 54702-1000

16127937R00110

Made in the USA
Charleston, SC
06 December 2012